Eating
in
Eden

Eating in Eden

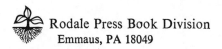

By Ruth Adams

The Nutritional Superiority
of "Primitive" Foods

Rodale Press Book Division
Emmaus, PA 18049

Printed in the United States of America

FIRST PRINTING—March 1976
PB-359

Library of Congress Cataloging in Publication Data

Adams, Ruth 1923–
  Eating in Eden.

  Bibliography: p.177
  Includes index.
  1. Nutrition. 2. Diet. 3. Food. I. Title.
TX353.A3 1975   641.1   75–32567
ISBN 0–87857–109–4

Contents

Introduction

What do the words "primitive diet" mean as they are used in this book? Can one call Imperial Rome "primitive" when it was a highly sophisticated society for many centuries? Is the ancient, world-famous cuisine of China "primitive" by any standard? Was the diet of Tudor England "primitive?" The Aztecs, Incas and Mayans had marvelously sophisticated cultures that endured for thousands of years. Were their diets primitive?

I have undertaken to define "primitive diet" as any diet, anywhere in the world, which did (or does) *not* consist in large part of highly refined foods, which make up about fifty percent of the average diet today in Western industrialized countries. In Imperial Rome there was no cereal industry, turning out puffed-up, sugary goodies to tempt children. There was no baking industry as we know it today. There were bakers who were generally also the people who milled the grain. They could, with great trouble, sift out some of the branny parts of the grain—but not very much, we suspect. In later times the bread eaten by almost everybody was wholegrain, heavy, tough, tasty. White bread, especially the superwhite, highly-refined, doughy, gummy stuff on supermarket shelves today was unknown and undreamed-of.

The earliest man we know of was what anthropologists call a "gatherer." He wandered, as raccoons, as reindeer and buffalo wander, looking for edible things—fruits, nuts, berries, roots, leaves, seeds. In his search he found many sources of animal food as well—grubs, insects, small mammals and birds, frogs, fish, shellfish, fish eggs, snails, turtles, birds' eggs and so on. So our ancient ancestors were never purely vegetarian.

By the time they discovered that weapons could be used to kill larger animals, they became "hunter-gatherers." Society changed. Migrations now were planned according to where the game was, as well as where there was food of vegetable origin. The greatest cause of rejoicing was the finding of a dead rhinoceros or hippopotamus, even half-rotted, for the whole tribe could then eat their way out of hunger for many days. Human beings still wandered. Over most of past history, for some two million years, our ancestors wandered the world, as "hunter-gatherers."

Sometimes they had enough food, at other times they must have been very hungry. In some parts of the planet, hunting and gathering were successful enough that human beings had some leisure time. Mostly they worked very hard to keep their stomachs full. People probably lived in small groups, so that hunters could cooperate in searching for game. Those who did not hunt, mostly the old folks, women and children, foraged for vegetable foods and probably ate them as they found them. Or they brought the treasures home to be shared and cooked. Except in cold regions perishable food could not be stored. It must be eaten at once, and it was, down to the very bones which were cracked, gnawed and cleaned of every bit of marrow, gristle and fat. *most must be cooked* *less common*

So for several million years, humankind ate meat, fish, birds' eggs, insects, fruits, roots, leaves, berries, nuts, seeds —and survived. Undoubtedly many people perished from infections, parasites, from unrecognized natural poisons in foods, from spoiled foods, from injuries, from genetic mutations which crippled them in some way. Undoubtedly, too, many people perished from vitamin deficiency diseases. Vitamin C was almost unavailable in northern countries for many months of the year. Many people died of scurvy. Rickets followed southern peoples as they migrated north, ignorant of the fact that sunshine falling on human skin creates vitamin D, which is essential for healthy bones. In the long northern winters there is little sunshine. One scientist has theorized that people living in northern countries are blonde because only blondes could survive there, since their skins admit more sunlight (hence vitamin D) than darker skins. In southern parts of the world, dark skins protect against too much sunshine and admit just enough vitamin D to prevent rickets. In lengthy, strenuous migrations northward, people crippled by rickets could not survive.

About 10,000 years ago some genius discovered that by planting seeds in one spot, grains could be grown, stored, and saved from year to year so that wandering was no longer necessary. Many human beings settled down in geographical areas where cereal grains would grow, and "civilization" began.

I used the word "genius" advisedly, for the ability to grasp the continuity of seed-to-plant-to-seed again must have required a great deal of serious agricultural research, if we want to describe it that way. Some experts think it may have been women who made the discovery since they were more or less in charge of the vegetable part of the diet. At any rate, somebody discovered that seeds could be buried in the earth, and would produce plants which would later produce more seeds. These seeds could be dried and stored and used by people until time to harvest the next year's crop.

Grant Allen, a Canadian philosopher, novelist and

science writer, theorizes that human beings may have discovered agriculture as a result of burial customs. They buried their dead with tools and food for use in the next world. The soil, disturbed for a grave, was good garden soil for seeds to sprout in. Observant people must have noticed that the seeds which had been buried with their loved one came up and produced more seeds. This may, Allen thinks, have been one reason for human and animal sacrifice. Perhaps ancient people thought that someone must die and be buried, in order for seeds to grow. So a sacrifice must be made at the beginning of each planting season. No one knows how correct this theory may be.

In any case, when human beings settled down to raise cereals as their staple foods, there was a great basic change in their diet. Cereals are starchy foods, generally speaking. Although they contain more protein than berries, fruits, or roots, they contain as much as 75 percent starch. So living creatures which had become accustomed over several million years to a generally high-protein diet changed over, rather rapidly, to a diet high in starch, when cereals became their main basic foods.

A group of very knowledgeable nutrition experts today believe firmly that the invention of agriculture and the consequent reliance on cereal foods as the basis of diet was the beginning, for mankind, of a group of disorders which these experts call "the diseases of civilization." They point out that such diseases were apparently unknown among earlier people who ate diets high in protein with considerably less starch.

How can such a theory be proved? There are still "primitive" people in remote corners of today's world who live as their ancestors lived, wandering, gathering and hunting. By studying the health of these people, we can perhaps find out whether, indeed, "civilized" human beings might avoid these "diseases of civilization" by returning, generally speaking, to a diet like the one eaten by our ancestors before civilization began.

The period of time during which human beings have been planting seeds and living in settled communities is but a moment in the aeons of time since life began on earth. Within the last hundred years or so—not even a fraction of a second in archeological time—another great change has come over the diet of "civilized" man. Millers learned how to refine cereals, taking out the "rough" part of the grain and making smooth, soft, silky, white flour, delightful to eat, easy to store and to make into bread, cakes, pies, and goodies.

At about the same time, technology was developed for refining sugar cane—that is, taking a huge, tough, 10-foot-high blade of grass, removing all the tough part and leaving only the sweet juice of the plant which is then refined into white sugar. Housewives, trying to relieve the monotony of winter meals where only gruel and a few dried vegetables might be available, seized eagerly on sugar, with which so many delicious things could be flavored. And human beings began to consume sugar in increasingly large amounts, until today the "civilized" countries are eating an average of more than 100 pounds per year for every individual. Since some people eat no sugar or very little (babies, diabetics, etc.) this means that many of the people who *do* eat sugar are eating far more than 100 pounds a year. Dieticians have discovered, with great surprise, that some people whose diets they analyze may be eating as much as 400 pounds of this concentrated sweet stuff in one year!

Nowhere in any "primitive" society can anybody obtain this much sugar to eat. So if researchers discover that the diseases of civilization are confined to those parts of the world where large amounts of refined cereal foods and white sugar are eaten, and are almost non-existent among primitive people who do not eat these foods, it seems fairly certain that these two foods may have a great deal to do with the soaring incidence of these diseases in the Western world.

What are these diseases? Obesity and overweight, diabetes, coronary heart conditions involving strokes and heart attacks, circulatory troubles including varicose veins, hemorrhoids, and hardening of the arteries, peptic ulcers, tooth decay, diverticulitis, colitis, constipation, hiatal hernia, gallstones, varicocele, and possibly many more conditions which are common in "civilized" countries.

Dr. John Yudkin of London University in England has written extensively on this subject, including one book on sugar entitled *Sweet and Dangerous.* Dr. T. L. Cleave and Dr. G. D. Campbell have written a fine book on *Diabetes, Coronary Thrombosis and the Saccharine Disease,* dealing with many of the disorders mentioned above in relation to "civilized" diet. Dr. Denis Burkitt of the Medical Research Council in London, Dr. Neil Painter of The Manor House Hospital, London, Dr. E. W. Pomare and K. W. Heaton of the Bristol Royal Infirmary, Bristol, England, are writing much significant material on the relation of our "fiber-free" diets to digestive diseases which are rapidly becoming very common causes of illness and death.

When our millers make white flour and processed cereals, they remove the fiber from the cereals and concentrate the fiberless starch. When our sugar companies refine sugar, they remove all the fiber of the sugar cane and concentrate the sugar.

In this book, I refer again and again to the health catastrophes that follow when long-established diet patterns are suddenly changed. The Ik in Africa rapidly starved to death when they were moved from their hunting territory to an agricultural land. Within a few years from the time Eskimos, American Indians or Africans leave their ancestral homes and diets, and move to town where they eat "civilized" diets, they rapidly fall prey to "the diseases of civilization."

Isn't it about time we realize what these two classifications of food—refined starches and sugars—are doing to us in the civilized countries—removed as we are by only 50 or 100 years from a much more primitive diet—the kind of diet, generally speaking, which is described on page after page of this book.

In general, it is safe to say that primitive people ate (and eat) anything that is edible in their environment. They work very hard to get it and to prepare it for eating. The Mexican housewife spends six hours every day preparing cornmeal for tortillas. The Balinese cook spends hours every day gathering coconut, cracking shells, digging out the meat, grating it, pounding it, making it into whatever dish she is preparing. Primitive Eskimo hunters endure unbelievable physical hardships to get food and bring it home. The women work constantly to prepare food and clothing from the few materials available.

So we must take into account one other aspect of our "civilized" lives which undoubtedly has much to do with our "diseases of civilization." *Technology has made us all but completely sedentary.* Getting dinner involves no more than opening the refrigerator, taking out the TV dinner and popping it into the oven. Eating an apple for most of us involves getting into the car, driving to the supermarket and buying a bag of apples.

Possibly if we were still eating the diets our ancient

ancestors ate, we might be able to get by, health-wise, on so little exercise. But, in addition to the sedentary nature of our lives, we now have added this further health complication— the consumption of vast amounts of concentrated starches and sugars which our digestive tracts are apparently unable to deal with in such large amounts. The result obviously must be overweight and obesity which, at present, afflict about half of all adults and about one-third of our children, who seem destined to go right on having weight problems as they grow older. It's quite possible they will also have to cope, somehow, with the co-existing diseases of civilization mentioned above.

I do not want to give the impression that our ancestors, and the few primitive groups of people still living in their ancestral way, are "noble savages," that their lives were or are a blissful idyll of innocence and languor. The Brothwells in their fine book, *Food in Antiquity,* describe some of the horrors earlier people faced, aside from cold, darkness and ignorance of even basic rules of hygiene.

In general, the hunter-gatherer peoples were less likely to face adverse health conditions than the early agricultural peoples. Severe malnutrition and vitamin and mineral deficiencies plagued early people in many parts of the world. Wars and frequent famines brought hunger and starvation. In one era the Nile did not perform its usual yearly flooding rite for seven years, so there were seven years of famine.

In England there were more than 200 famines between 10 A.D. and 1850. In China there were 1,800 famines between 100 B.C. and 1910 A.D. The Aztecs suffered severe famines from 1451 to 1456. Rusts and other diseases afflicted the cereal crops from the earliest days of agriculture. Even today, losses from disease on a worldwide scale may be as high as 60 percent of the crop. In earlier days every loss affected the daily food of millions of people. Stock animals died of anthrax and pox.

Scurvy, the disease of vitamin C deficiency, killed untold millions of people: sailors on long voyages, soldiers on long marches, citizens cooped up in cities under seige. Pellagra, caused by lack of a B vitamin, undoubtedly made inroads wherever corn was the basis of the diet, with no wise addition of other foods which would complement the vitamin and amino acid deficiency in corn. Goiter, caused by lack of iodine, plagued people living in far inland regions or high mountains.

Infant mortality was high because it was difficult to devise nutritional foods for weaning infants and because hygiene was unknown. Children whose mothers died in childbirth were almost certainly doomed, for there was no way to feed infants but the human breast. Some foods contain toxic elements which become dangerous when these foods make up the main items of diet. Those ancient people had to learn by trial and error, and error must often have meant unexplained death.

Parasites preyed on human beings. Wildlife is almost universally infested with worms or grubs of one kind or another. Food from such animals, eaten raw, poses a serious threat to the health of the human being who eats it. Noxious insects, against which there was no defense, must have caused a great deal of disease, especially in tropical countries. Ergot is a fungus disease of cereals which causes madness and hallucinations in people who eat the affected grains. How could our ancestors have known this was the cause?

But, in the light of all this, isn't it astonishing that there is so little reference in ancient history to heart attacks, strokes, constipation, diabetes, varicose veins, tooth decay, gallstones, peptic ulcers? It is not appropriate or accurate to explain this by saying that primitive people just never lived long enough to reach the age at which such diseases attack. Today teenagers are falling prey to these disorders. Babies have tooth decay. The degenerative disease cancer is the chief cause of death from disease among children. Young adults in the very prime of life are victims of one or several of these degenerative disorders. Isn't it about time we wiped out these diet-related diseases, now that we have done a fairly good job of controlling infectious diseases and parasites, we understand the importance of vitamins and minerals, and we have established the basis of good general hygiene throughout the industrialized world?

If we cannot manage a world-wide revolution in thinking about refined food, at least it seems possible to achieve a great deal in the way of personal and family health by looking at the foods which kept primitive people healthy, in spite of the terrible threats they faced from famines, infectious disease, parasites, natural poisons in food, and other illnesses.

Recent statistics on population and food seem to indicate that we are rapidly approaching a time when even the rich Western nations will have to scramble for food, if they share even a small part of their harvests with their impoverished brethren in The Third World, whose numbers are exploding at a frightful rate, while literally hundreds of million of them face hunger, malnutrition and starvation right now.

Wouldn't it be wise, before this time of austerity takes us by surprise, to know something of the ways in which our ancestors pieced out their meals, without ever tasting a TV dinner or a chocolate bar? Wouldn't it be smart to know the best way, apparently, to avoid malnutrition, even when food is scarce—namely, to make every mouthful count, nutritionally, so that not one cent of money or one moment of time or one precious crumb of garden soil is wasted on foods that do not nourish, but instead bring chronic disease?

In the process, of course, it's possible we may develop into more likeable and successful human beings. Marston Bates says, in *Where Winter Never Comes,* "The resources of the world for a cabbage butterfly can be studied in terms of the availability of cabbages; for an owl, in terms of field mice and nesting sites. The economy of food-gathering man was probably not much more complicated, being rather like that of any omnivorous mammal—a raccoon, for instance. But with the acquisition and development of culture, all of this changed and the economy of man started gaining complexity, at first slowly, but later with the specialization and diversification of civilization, at a dizzily increasing rate. To-day's results often seem to be an economy that is beyond the comprehension of any of its human creators; or at least, quite plainly beyond my comprehension. . . .

"A few peoples apparently have never taken up with any of these insidious methods of food producing; we find them today in a food-gathering culture that seems not un-like the culture that probably characterized all of mankind 15,000 or 20,000 years ago. We call such people 'backward' —but maybe they are the cleverest of all in having managed to avoid, through all of these millenia, those first fatal steps toward the primrose-lined, ambition-greased chute of civilization."

That is what this book is about. Read it in good health.

The Near-Perfect
Nutritional State of
Primitive People

A classic book *Nutrition and Physical Degeneration* has been re-issued as perhaps the most convincing testament we could have of the blessings of natural foods and the physical blight visited upon those people who succumb to the attraction of modern processed and refined foods. Its author, Dr. Weston Price, a dentist with a string of honors after his name, along with a list of learned societies to which he belonged, wrote, in 1939, the story of his travels to the far corners of the world to study the teeth and general health of so-called "primitive" people.

Dr. Price and his wife travelled to Africa, New Zealand, Australia, South America, Polynesia and isolated corners of Switzerland. They visited with Alaskan Eskimos, American Indians and Gaelic people living on faraway islands. Considering what the difficulties of the trip must have been at that time, we all owe Dr. Price a profound debt of gratitude for his courage and fortitude and the vast amount of illustrative material he brought back. His book rapidly became a classic and many printings were made.

One could almost say that the photographs tell the story. Indeed, just glancing through the book one sees massive evidence of what civilization, with its refined and processed foods, has brought to these more primitive people. There are pictures of decayed teeth, deformed dental arches and facial structure, along with other bodily deformities of many kinds. These are present in people eating diets in which refined foods play a large part. In people who live in the same communities or nearby communities, but do not eat these "civilized" foods, the photos show magnificent physiques, flawless carriage and bone structures, and near perfect teeth.

Dr. Price did not start out with any preconceived notion of what he might find. What he did find is staggering in its implications for the "civilized" nations. For he brought back convincing evidence that it takes apparently only one generation of wrong eating to destroy a family heritage of perfect teeth and bone structure, jaw structure, jaw alignment and dental arches. On page after page, one sees contrasting pictures of members of the same family, one who continued to eat his "native," ancestral diet, the other who switched to refined foods. The first photo shows perfect teeth and bone structure. His brother or sister eating "modern" food has already developed such bad teeth that half of them are rotted away.

The content of the ancestral diet didn't seem to matter very much, so long as there was enough complete protein, vitamins and minerals. And no refined carbohydrates. Swiss children and their ancestors lived all their lives on almost nothing but rye bread, milk and cheese. Some of the children ate roasted rye grains instead of bread. Their young cousins, living in parts of the same areas where plenty of pastries, candies and jams were available, had up to 30 percent of their teeth destroyed by decay.

Eskimo children, living on salmon, seal meat and other food from animal sources, had no tooth decay, perfect dental arches, no crowding of teeth. Their fathers were able to

2

carry packs weighing 100 pounds *in their teeth*. But relatives, living in areas where "store grub" was available opened their mouths, at Dr. Price's invitation, to show rows of decayed and rotted teeth, deformities of arches, teeth crowded into mouths too small to contain them. "In many districts," says Dr. Price, "dental service cannot be obtained and suffering is acute and prolonged."

In the Hebrides Islands, Gaelic people living as their ancestors had lived for many years, ate oats, barley, fish and seafood of all kinds. Describing the women, all with perfect teeth, working at their fish-cleaning benches, Dr. Price says, "It would be difficult to find examples of womanhood combining a higher degree of physical perfection and more exalted ideals than these weather-hardened toilers. . . . One marvels at their gentleness, refinement and sweetness of character."

At the fringe of civilization, however, Dr. Price encountered in a seaport town about one hundred inhabitants, 25 of whom were already wearing dentures, another 25 of whom should have been wearing them. Stores in this part of the Islands were jammed with white flour and white sugar products: cakes, white bread, jams, jellies, candies, sweetened fruit juices. In one home two young brothers sat at the same table. One was eating oatmeal, oatcake and sea foods. He had excellent teeth. His brother, across the table, insisted on having white bread, jam, highly sweetened coffee and chocolates. His teeth were nearly gone. His father was deeply concerned with how hard it was to get him up in the morning.

On page after page the same story is told. Describing the havoc wrought by refined foods among the Melanesians in New Caledonia and the Fiji Isles, Dr. Price tells us in one poignant sentence, "Toothache is the only cause of suicide." But among the primitive peoples of the island, Dr. Price could find almost no decay. These people ate seafood, along

3

with plants and fruits. In their "civilized" brothers, eating white flour products, sugar, canned foods and polished rice, general incidence of tooth decay was 30 percent of all teeth.

Dr. Price, deeply involved in the study of anthropology, shows photographs of ancient skulls found in Peruvian ruins. In a study of almost 1,300 skulls from ancient civilizations of Peru, he tells us he did not find a single skull with deformity of the dental arches. He says also that up to 75 percent of all individuals in some parts of the United States have such deformities.

In the final chapters of the book, Dr. Price covers the physical and mental deterioration that accompanies these tragic deformities of jaws and dental arches. He gives statistics on delinquents and criminals. He describes his own examinations of people housed in prisons and schools for delinquents. There was ample evidence of serious nutritional deficiency in early childhood and before birth, demonstrated by bone structure and jaw development. Mental deficiency accompanied the physical disorders.

One gradually begins to understand the word "degeneration" in the title of Dr. Price's book. He means, simply, the degeneration of the human race which is rapidly overtaking us, on account of the poor nutritional state we are in, because so much of our diet consists of denatured foods which do not contain the basic nutritional building blocks we need to survive, as a race of people.

Dr. Price discusses the deterioration of soils the world over, as we take crop after crop off the earth without replacing anything. "The complacency with which the masses of the people as well as the politicians view our trend," he says, "is not unlike the drifting of a merry party in the rapids above a great cataract. There seems to be no appropriate sense of impending doom."

In a beautiful final chapter Dr. Price suggests how we

4

might apply primitive wisdom to solve some of our modern problems. He describes traditional ways of handling marriage, childbirth, adolescence and old age. He tells us how primitive people manage their agriculture and care for their soil. He tells us that a basic understanding of the primitive way of doing things is essential "for stemming the tide of our progressive breakdown and also for our return to harmony with Nature's laws, since life in its fullness is Nature obeyed."

Dr. Price's monumental work is now 33 years old. Everything he foresaw in the way of degeneration is proceeding so rapidly that many philosophers see no way out of the dilemma we are in. Practically all the really primitive people he saw, studied and photographed have long since succumbed to the lure of processed foods and suffer from the same disorders that plague us in this country: tooth decay, digestive tract diseases, heart and artery problems, obesity, overweight and so on. There are few places left today where anyone can go to find people still untouched by "civilization."

What have we learned? Due to this early work of Dr. Price and the valuable work of other early nutrition experts like Dr. Clive McCay of Cornell University, many of us have learned that we cannot be healthy and cannot have healthy children when we exist on diets consisting in large part of foods that have been ruined by being stripped of almost everything that renders them valuable as food. We know that all breads and cereals must be truly wholegrain. We know that we must abjure forever the use of sugar and any and all foods and beverages made with it.

Aside from this, it's not too important what we eat, so long as we get enough complete protein, vitamins and minerals. As Dr. Price showed clearly, diets consisting almost entirely of food of animal origin—meat, fish, milk, cheese,

5

poultry—sustained and nourished in good health many of the primitive people he visited. And, so long as complete protein was available, much greater reliance on foods of vegetable origin—grains, seeds, nuts, fruits and vegetables —seemed to produce abundant health in those societies where food of animal origin was scarce.

But in both the meat-eating and the vegetarian societies, the changeover to a largely "civilized" diet of which perhaps half or more of every meal consisted of refined carbohydrates, brought catastrophe *within the short space of one generation.* This is due, apparently, to the disarrangement of bodily mechanisms produced by these refined foods which are, remember, quite new to human experience.

As you will see in the following pages, no human being, over the past two million years, ever had access to such "foods" as these. Primitive man ate whole foods, simply because he had no way to refine or process them completely enough to remove most of their essential nutrients. And that is precisely what the food technologists of our giant food industry have done today.

If you are looking for the perfect diet, then, so far as good nutrition and good health are concerned, look no farther. Just return to the kind of meals your ancestors survived on for millions of years. How do you accomplish that? Remove from your shopping lists, your kitchen shelves and your dining table all processed and refined foods. This includes everything that contains white flour and white sugar as well as those cold cereals in the gaudy boxes which crowd the long shelves at the supermarket.

What is left for you to eat will nourish you completely. Primitive people ate everything in their environment that was edible. So cut loose! Eat as wide a variety as possible of meat, poultry, fish, shellfish, eggs, dairy products, fruits, vegetables, seeds, nuts, wholegrain cereals and breads.

Chapter
2

Most Europeans Ate "Primitive" Diets up to the Twentieth Century

Pompeii, the ancient city in Italy, was destroyed by the eruption of Vesuvius in 79 A.D. After studying the graffiti and inscriptions still on the walls, archeologists have hazarded educated guesses as to some of the foods which were available in Pompeii at that time. Helen Tanzer tells us in *The Common People of Pompeii* that gourmet food was every bit as important to the early Italians as it is to us today. But their ideas of gourmet fare differed somewhat from ours.

Food, both raw and cooked, was sold in the streets of Pompeii, in shops and in stands, as well as from trays carried by itinerant vendors. One scene, which archeologists found painted on a wall, shows a vendor dipping something hot from a large vessel and selling it to his customers, while a young woman sells vegetables and figs. In another scene, an old peddler has fallen asleep. A passerby is tapping his shoulder to wake him, so he can serve the two customers who are holding out bowls for what appears to be fried food.

In the markets which specialized in fruits and vegetables there were cherries, dates and lupines (seeds of the lupine flower which were eaten like beans). Italians in New York in the 1930's still ate lupines, says Tanzer, first soaking them in water to remove the bitterness.

Garlic, wheat, barley and bran (*furfur*) were eaten, as were chicken and pork, cheese from goat or sheep milk, mustard, leeks and a sauce called *garum* for which Pompeii was famous. The sauce, also called *liquamen,* was made in Pompeii from the intestines of a Spanish mackerel, heavily salted, exposed to the sun and stirred every day for several months. The vats were covered at night to protect them from the rain. The intestines gradually dissolved and the liquid—*garum*—was drained off. It was distributed in small pitchers.

Another recipe calls for sprats, anchovies or mackerel, with two pints of salt to a peck of fish. This mixture stood in the sun for two or three months, was stirred occasionally, and old wine was added sometimes. The finished sauce was a clear, golden liquid which kept well and had a salty, slightly fishy or cheesy taste. It was used in most dishes in Rome.

The use of herbs, sauces and spices in Roman food boggles the mind. In the cookbook compiled by Apicius, a Roman gourmet, a recipe for roast meat lists as ingredients ¼ ounce of each of the following: pepper, lovage, parsley, celery seed, dill, asafetida root, *cyperus* (umbrella plant), caraway, cumin, ginger, pyrethrum, 1¼ pints of *liquamen* or *garum* and 2½ ounces of olive oil. Since Roman dinner parties usually consisted of nine people, the roast, drowned in such a sauce, might be expected to serve each diner five or six tablespoons of this very spicy sauce.

We do not know what early Roman food actually tasted like since there is no way of knowing how much fat their meat had, how stale or fresh the spices and herbs were, or how much they were used to conceal the taste of spoiled or rancid food, for there was no refrigeration.

The Romans used lead and pewter which contained lead, to make cooking utensils and jars in which food was stored. Wine merchants often added to their wine a preservative syrup which had been boiled in lead-lined pots. One symptom of chronic lead poisoning is lack of appetite and a metallic taste in the mouth. Some modern scientists believe that the people of the Roman Empire suffered from chronic lead poisoning which may have been the chief cause of the Empire's decline and fall.

Lack of appetite and a strong, unpleasant taste in the mouth might make strong, pungent, spicy sauces appealing. The rich Romans used these hot sauces chiefly on meat and fish dishes which dilute the sauce hardly at all, since they do not absorb much of it. Poor people, who had more starchy food as the basis for their meals, found such sauces much less pungent since the rice, pasta or gruel absorb sauces and dilute their strong flavors.

The barbarians who conquered Rome in the fifth century demanded as tribute not only lands, subsidies and military titles for their chief, but three thousand pounds of pepper as well!

A Roman senator, coming home to dinner might have found on the table a stew of diced pork shoulder simmered in a wine sauce, with shallots, mint, dill and apricots, or the same cut of pork combined with apples and leeks and spiced with cumin and coriander. In winter, dinner might well have been baked beans with bits of chicken, sausages, leeks and fennel, or a patina of soles seasoned with oregano and lovage.

According to Betty Wason in *Cooks, Gluttons and Gourmets,* even vegetables were lavishly seasoned with oregano or blended with eggs into a patina or simmered in oil with herbs, or pureed and dressed with mustard sauce. Cabbage was cooked in wine, flavored with cumin and mint, garnished with chopped, fresh olives.

Sweets were fairly simple, she tells us. She found few

recipes for desserts in the book of recipes collected by Apicius. One for cheesecake turned out to be just a sweetened custard of milk and eggs. Another dessert was bread, soaked in milk, fried, then topped with honey—much like what we call "French toast."

Apicius, whom Wason calls "the Fanny Farmer of Imperial Rome," was such a determined gourmet that he killed himself after one splendid banquet on which he had spent much of his fortune, since there was no chance he would be able to afford such luxurious, expensive food in the future.

The *Journal of the American Medical Association* for December 11, 1967, published a menu found in a noble house in the ruins of Pompeii. It consisted of a first course of sea urchins, several kinds of oysters, larks, a hen pullet with asparagus, mussels, white and black sea tulips. The second course included assorted shellfish, cutlets of kid and boar meat, chicken pie, roasted songbirds with asparagus sauce. In the third course, there was a wild boar's head, the teats of a sow, breasts and necks of roast ducks, wild duck fricasseed, roast hare, roasted Phrygian chickens, starch cream (perhaps a kind of custard) and cakes. Honey and dates were usually used for sweetening.

As one might expect, none of these foods was available for the poor Romans, of whom there seem to have been an astonishingly large number, since almost one-third of the city's population was at one time "on relief." That is, they were getting free grain from the Emperor. Poor Romans ate mostly bread, gruels made of grain, porridge made of millet, plus olives, raw beans, figs and cheese.

During the Middle Ages, frumenty was perhaps the food most widely used in Europe. This consisted of husked wheat soaked in hot water for 24 hours until it turned into a kind of milky jelly. It could be eaten cold with honey, or hot with whatever was available in the way of bits of meat, fish or vegetables.

The pot which hung over the fire in rich and poor homes alike bubbled most of the time, probably, summer and winter. Into it went whatever meat was available—salt pork, a rabbit or a hen. Most days whatever came out of the pot was dinner, as well as breakfast and lunch, along with bread or frumenty. Pease porridges (like our cornmeal mush) were made of dried beans, peas or lentils and they went well with salt pork. They could be used hot or cold or, as the old rhyme says, "in the pot, nine days old."

An early English cookbook gives this recipe for rabbit (*cony*) stew: "*Take a cony and perboyle it a little, then take a good handful of persely and a few sweete hearbes, the yolke of iii hard egges, chop them altogether then put in pepper and a few currantes and fill the Contes bellieful of Butter then psiche her head betweene her hinder legges and brake her not and put her into a faire earthern pot with mutton broth and the rest of the stuffe roll it round and put it withall and so boyle them well together and serve it with soppes.*"

In Tudor England (1485–1600, approximately) the gentry dined at 11 in the morning, eating and talking until perhaps two or three in the afternoon, then sitting down again for supper at six. Merchants and farmers dined at noon and supped at seven or eight. Farmers had simple fare: meat, bacon, poultry, fruit, cheese, butter, eggs. Poor people ate, according to one contemporary writer, "the refuse meat, scraps and parings such as a dog would scarse eat sometimes," and, "The poore with us woulde think themselves happy if they might have a messe of potage or the scraps that come from the rich mens table, two or three hours after they begin their dinner or supper, and to have the same given them at the door. . . ."

11

Rich men might eat *at one meal,* we are told, beef, mutton, veal, lamb, kid, pork, cony, capon, pig, "or so many of these as the season yieldeth, but also some portions of the red or fallow deer, beside great variety of fish and wild fowl." Of course, there were always many guests, servants and retainers to be fed, "and what is left over to the poore."

When Queen Elizabeth the First and the large party that must have travelled with her visited Lord North's house for three days in 1577, we are told that provisions for those three days added up to: 17½ quarters (of a bushel, presumably) of wheat for bread, 67 sheep, 34 pigs, four stags and 16 bucks, 1,200 chickens, 363 capons, 33 geese, 6 "turkies," 237 pigeons and quantities of partridges, snipe, quail, and "all other kinds of birds including gulls," a cartload and two horseloads of oysters, fish in endless variety, 2,500 eggs, 430 pounds of butter. What must have been involved in preparing such a feast in a kitchen where cooking was done on spits over an open fire or in huge kettles bubbling away!

One important point is that all the foods mentioned above are protein and fat foods. There is almost no carbohydrate. But rich people used spices and some sugar, as well. Nine out of ten recipes contained spices in what seem to us extremely large amounts. Sugar was very expensive, hence available only for the rich. An article in *The Journal of the American Dental Association* comments on the results of heavy sugar eating, in regard to Queen Elizabeth the First of England. It seems that throughout the Queen's 45-year reign, she suffered from decayed and diseased teeth which tormented her night and day and may have been responsible for her death.

Her permanent teeth had trouble erupting. She went on to suffer from rampant tooth decay, chronic toothache, facial pains and gum deterioration. Often these conditions

12

became so noticeable that state visitors could not help but comment. Many state occasions had to be postponed because the Queen was suffering from an intense toothache.

On one occasion when her pain had endured many days and nights, the doctors recommended pulling the decayed tooth. Elizabeth could not face the pain. Anesthesia was unknown. Teeth were usually pulled by barbers who accompanied clowns and jugglers to fairs where they pulled the teeth of fairgoers. A good friend of the Queen's, the Bishop of London (an old man) offered to have one of his teeth pulled to show her that the pain was endurable.

Contemporary descriptions of the Queen, commenting on her beauty, her fine posture and her gracious ways, could not avoid adding that her teeth were "yellow" or "black" and many of them were missing. In her painted portraits, she is never pictured smiling and, in later years, the deterioration of her mouth structure is apparent; her oval face shortened and eventually she appeared jowly and heavy.

At that time there were no ways to replace teeth, or to treat toothache except with herbs and potions. So the richest and most glamorous queen in Western history had to live out her life in pain, not only physical, but psychological, for she was vain and could not help but know that the rotten teeth spoiled her looks.

There seems to be no doubt what caused the Queen's condition. "Her teeth are black (a defect the British seem subject to, from their too great use of sugar)," said a contemporary commentator. A modern historian tells us that Elizabeth was inordinately fond of sweets and carried some kind of confection with her wherever she went. Elizabeth's death is believed to have been caused by a septic condition of her mouth—an infected tooth.

The poor people of England, who could not afford sweets, were also condemned by poverty to eat coarse brown bread, which gave their teeth, gums and jaws a lot of excellent, healthful exercise. Other chewy foods like beans and lentils also helped to keep their teeth healthy. But the noblemen and their queen ate whiter bread and sugar which, said a contemporary historian, "heateth the blood, rotteth the teeth, maketh them look black."

However, down through all the ages up to the present century, sugar was used mostly as a spice or a medicine because of its high price. No one, not even a queen, could have eaten 100 pounds of sugar or more in a year. But this is the average amount eaten today, even by very poor people in the industrialized world.

Drummond and Wilbraham in *The Englishman's Food,* give the best idea of how English people ate through the centuries and what their nutritional problems were. The book has chapters on rickets, scurvy, tooth decay, bone growth, constipation, vitamin deficiency and food adulteration. It details what people actually ate from day to day—poor people and rich people alike.

In medieval and Tudor Europe, Drummond and Wilbraham tell us, the diet of the peasant consisted of coarse black bread made of *maslin* (mixed wheat and rye), barley, rye or bean flour, milk, cheese, eggs (which were plentiful) and sometimes bacon or poultry. He drank whey, buttermilk or water and sometimes ale. He had little meat except when he managed some successful poaching. Even so, the diet was high in protein, minerals and B vitamins, but almost completely lacking in vitamin A and vitamin C. Of course, famine stalked him, for a poor harvest, too much or too little rain, could mean the difference between a fairly comfortable diet and starvation.

Rich people ate meat of all kinds, fowl, fish and game, and drank fine wines, ale, beer and cider. Occasionally there are records of greens and beets, leeks and garlic being

14

eaten, but seldom fresh fruits or other vegetables.

The townspeople ate breakfast about six or seven in the morning. It consisted of bread, salted or pickled herrings, cold meat, pottage, cheese and ale. The midday meal included roast meats, pies, stews or soups, bread, cheese and ale. Around five or six P.M. supper came to the table as cold meat, cheese and bread, served with ale or wine. The only vegetables used in quantities were onions, or occasionally cabbages.

Assessing a peasant's diet in England up to medieval times, Drummond and Wilbraham tell us it was far better than many modern diets, with the exception of its lack of vitamin C. By the end of winter, when fresh foods were unavailable, most of the country people must have been in a "pre-scorbutic" state—that is, verging on scurvy, the disease of vitamin C deficiency. In any family unable to produce or buy milk and eggs, vitamin A deficiency was also a real threat. Cows fed dried hay all winter give little vitamin A in their milk. Eggs from hens eating feed which contains no vitamin A contain little of the vitamin. So early spring was a dangerous time for many reasons.

Wealthy Englishmen got an estimated 200 to 300 grams of animal protein daily. The official U.S. recommendation for adults is 46 to 56 grams daily. Kidney stones were common among English gentry of this period. Drummond and Wilbraham suggest that the reason was lack of vitamin A, combined with a great deal of calcium from milk.

Scurvy was common until the 18th century, not only among sailors on long trips, soldiers on long marches and whole populations besieged in cities, but among country and town people who did not get enough fresh fruits or vegetables. Doctors wrangled and debated over the cause of scurvy, thinking up the most outlandish reasons for this

15

plague. Several books appeared showing that merely by including fresh fruits and vegetables at mealtime, doctors could cure and prevent scurvy. They were mostly (characteristically) ignored by official medicine, which thought scurvy might be caused by eating salt, for of course much of the meat was salted to preserve it.

In 1745 daily rations of the Royal Navy went like this: biscuits, beer, beef, pork, dried peas, oatmeal, butter and cheese. No vitamin C there and precious little vitamin A. By 1762 children in English orphanages and schools were eating bread, butter, gruel, milk, porridge, roast beef and "greens," potatoes, parsnips, mutton and rice pudding. We are not told what the "greens" were. Cooked, they would probably contain few vitamins. If it was cabbage, that one food alone might have sufficed to keep scurvy at bay.

Rickets, caused by deficiency of vitamin D, calcium and/or phosphorus, was common among the poor in England in the 17th and 18th centuries. Doctors there and elsewhere had no idea what caused it. The first recorded trial of cod liver oil for rheumatism was made in 1782 in Manchester. The doctors immediately bought fifty gallons of this nauseating stuff and forced it down the unwilling throats of their patients who were suffering from rheumatism, rickets, joint afflictions resulting from tuberculosis and almost any other disease involving bones and joints. The rickets patients improved at once, for fish liver oil is the most abundant source of vitamin D. The only other dependable source is sunlight. But England, by this time, was getting involved in the industrial revolution. Most of her poorest urban citizens lived in dark, dank alleys where the sun never shone for many months of the year.

In 1890 in England, the roller mill replaced the ancient methods of grinding flour between two huge millstones. The new milling methods removed most of the bran and wheat germ in which the B vitamins, iron and many other minerals are concentrated.

According to Drummond and Wilbraham, "The poor were most affected because they depended to a greater extent than the rich on bread and could not afford to buy other foods which might have readjusted this balance. The gravely deficient 'poverty' diet of England which persisted . . . from about 1890 . . . was responsible for a marked deficiency in the physique and physical efficiency of much of the community."

They go on to remind us that these dietary deficiencies were not serious enough to cause beriberi, though undoubtedly they did cause much nutritional anemia. Nutrition experts are certain that the roller mills and their methods of grinding flour affected the peoples' health adversely, but it is impossible to prove these facts. "Unfortunately it takes a long time to discover what minor ills and ailments have their origin in relatively mild deficiencies," they say. And much of modern nutritional science is proving the truth of that statement.

When Dr. Price visited the Isle of Harris in the 1930's he marvelled at the near-perfect teeth of the people there who were still living on their ancestral diets which consisted mostly of whole oats prepared in various ways, plus the wealth of seafood that is always available.

In the little remote town of Scalpay, he could find only one decayed tooth in the 100 children he examined. These children were eating fish and shellfish, oatmeal and oat cake, and not much more. Only ten miles away was the town of Tarbert where Harris Tweeds are exported to the world. Ships called at the port frequently and brought "civilization's" foods to the townspeople: white baker's bread, jams, marmalades, canned foods and all the other goodies we know so well. Dr. Price found an average of 32.4 decayed teeth per child among 100 of these children. One young man whose mouth was full of decayed teeth told Dr. Price he would have to travel 60 miles to the nearest dentist and have all his teeth pulled. ʿ hat was a common experience at Tarbert, he said. Dr. Price comments on the contrasting bone structure of faces in these two towns. In Tarbert the effects of a diet high in sugar and processed cereals were revealed in narrow dental arches, pinched faces and many degenerative diseases (such as tuberculosis) which had been hitherto unknown among the islanders.

Comparing the minerals in the diets of people living on the Outer Hebrides Islands, Dr. Price found that the traditional diet contained 2.1 times more calcium, 2.3 times more phosphorus, 1.3 times more magnesium and twice as much iron, as well as 10 times more of the fat soluble vitamins.

In the 1930's native people who lived high in the Alps were very isolated from "civilization." Dr. Price recounts his visit to one such locality, the Loetschental Valley. He found the same situation he had found in the New Hebrides. The Swiss children who were still eating the traditional diet, mostly homemade rye bread and homemade cheese, had near-perfect teeth. In another village, not far away, where a railroad had been built, children's teeth were decaying at a rapid rate. The stores were filled with candy, jam, sugar, syrup and highly sweetened canned fruits.

Dr. Price says that the people on traditional diets ate rye bread and dairy products almost exclusively, plus vegetables, fresh in summer and stored for winter. They had meat perhaps once a week. His analysis of the dairy products through a series of years showed the vitamin content to be much higher than the average throughout the world for similar foods through all seasons. The milk was produced from green pastures and stored green hay with a large content of chlorophyll, the green coloring matter in plants.

Comparing the native diet of the Swiss mountaineers in remote regions with the modern diet which displaced it in some areas, Dr. Price found that the traditional diet contained 3.7 times more calcium, 2.2 times more phosphorus, 2.5 times more magnesium, 3.1 times more iron and ten times more of the fat soluble vitamins.

Today in all of Western Europe, the "primitive" diet of the old-time Europeans has disappeared. Everybody eats just about what we eat in this country, with sugar and refined starches making up about half the calorie content of every day's meals. Dr. Price's work is being continued by a group of determined, vociferous, well-informed British scientists, several of whom recently came to Washington to testify at a Senate Committee hearing: Dr. John Yudkin, Dr. T. L. Cleave and Dr. G. D. Campbell. All of them deplore the use of refined carbohydrates and refined sugar.

In 1964, Dr. Yudkin's book *The Complete Slimmer* introduced the low carbohydrate diet for taking off weight. His recent book, *Sweet and Dangerous,* gives the hair-raising facts about the pernicious role sugar plays in modern diets and the terrible damage it is doing, especially to our children who have never known any time when cokes, candy, chewing gum and other sugary snacks were not available almost everywhere they go.

Dr. Cleave and Dr. Campbell have accumulated impressive statistics on the almost total absence of the "disease of civilization" among the primitive peoples left in the world who are still eating their traditional diets. The "civilization" diseases on which these two physician researchers have collected statistics are varicose veins, obesity, heart disease and other circulatory troubles, diabetes, tooth decay, hemorrhoids, peptic ulcer and many colonic conditions.

More recently, another group of British physicians is

pelting the medical establishment with facts on the harm we are doing to our health when we remove the fiber from sugar cane and cereals. This takes place during the refining process, when protein, vitamins and minerals are also removed. Dr. Denis Burkitt, Dr. Neil Painter, Dr. E. W. Pomare and Dr. K. W. Heaton are turning up significant relationships between bran (the fiber in wholegrain cereals) and the health of the entire digestive tract. They claim that the removal of this important source of roughage is involved in almost every digestive disease we suffer from: hiatal hernia, diverticulitis and diverticulosis, colitis, constipation, gallstones, and, almost certainly, cancer of the colon, the incidence of which is rising sharply in all Western industrialized nations.

Reluctantly, it seems, American medicine is taking at least token recognition of these facts. Once in a while an article on sugar, bran or processed cereals appears in the pages of an American medical journal among all the gaudy ads for drugs. The possibility seems remote of eventually getting complete recognition from either official medicine or the public health branches of the federal government that *this* is the diet revolution essential for immeasurably improving the health of the American people: the removal of all these offending carbohydrates from our diet. This means, in essence, a return to "primitive" diet—that is, meat, poultry, fish, shellfish, eggs, dairy products, fruits, vegetables, whole seeds, nuts, and only wholegrain cereals and breads. The way you cook or do not cook them, the way you combine them at mealtime, seem not to be important. What's important is the natural, unprocessed quality of the food itself.

Hunza and Other Shangri-Las

Remember "The Healthy Hunzas?" How are they faring these days? Have the past stories about their fabled health and longevity proved false? Has "civilization" with its attendant threats to good health, reached them at last and destroyed this Shangri-la where vigor and longevity are far more common than in most countries? A recent expedition to that remote mountain fastness seems to show that the same good sense and good management prevail among the Hunzas. They can still be called "The Healthy Hunzas."

In case you are not familiar with Hunza, the first reports came from Sir Robert McCarrison, a British physician who was a regimental officer in this part of the world in the early days of this century. Part of his territory was Gilgit in which the tiny nation of Hunza was located. It is in a corner of present-day Pakistan, high in the Karakorums Mountains, close to China and the Soviet Union.

Sir Robert contributed much in the way of nutritional experiments and pointed out, even at that early era of nutritional science, that we damage our health when we eat refined and processed carbohydrates. He became engrossed in studying the health of the Hunza people. He reported unequivocally that, in all the time he treated the Hunza people, he never saw a case of digestive disease or gastric or duodenal ulcer, appendicitis, cancer, mucus colitis. He said that disorders of the digestive region were simply unknown and "their buoyant abdominal health has, since my return to the West, provided a remarkable contrast with the dyspeptic and colonic lamentations of our highly civilized communities."

Since the time of Sir Robert, many other observers have reported on the Hunzas and speculated on why they are almost entirely free from many diseases which take a massive toll in "civilized" countries. J. I. Rodale wrote an early book, *The Healthy Hunzas.* Dr. Allen E. Banik, an optometrist, went to Hunza, sponsored by the Art Linkletter Program in 1958 and wrote a book about his trip, *Hunza Land.* Renee Taylor wrote a book in 1964 about her trip to Hunza. John H. Tobe told of his Hunza trip in a book called *Hunza: Adventures in a Land of Paradise.* In 1974 Senator Charles Percy visited Hunza as part of his work with the Senate Special Committee on Aging.

A professional man, specializing in gerontology (the care of old people) reported on Hunza recently in several professional journals. Alexander Leaf, M.D., Chief of Medical Services at Massachusetts General Hospital and Jackson, Professor of Clinical Medicine at Harvard Medical School, went to Hunza sponsored by the National Geographic Society. He visited other "pockets of longevity" as well and wrote fascinating reports on his trip in *The National Geographic Magazine,* January, 1973 and in *Nutrition Today,* September/October, 1973.

Dr. Leaf had some difficulty determining the age of the old people he talked to in Hunza, since there is no written language there and no birth records are kept. But their remembrances of historical facts, the ages of their children, grandchildren and great grandchildren all help to verify their ages. The oldest man in Hunza, according to Dr. Leaf, is Tulah Beg, who is 110. Another is 105. In *Nutrition Today* we see a photograph of eight old men waiting to see Dr. Leaf. Their ages range from 70 to 93. They are all active and interested in life.

Says Dr. Leaf, "The geography of Hunza requires everyone to work hard to eke out a living from the sparse terraces. In spite of (or because of) the primitive conditions, one sees an unusual number of vigorous elderly men and women agilely climbing up and down the steep slopes that line the habitable valley of these mountain dwellers." Dr. Leaf is not talking here of mountains as we think of them in our country. The Hunza valley is surrounded by mountain peaks over 20,000 feet high, with the highest, Rokaposhi, rearing its snow-capped head to 25,000 feet. Hunza garden plots are all on terraced hillsides, every stone of which was carried by hand to form the walls which hold the thin soil from sliding down the mountainside.

Dr. Leaf tells us that the diet of the Hunzas is sparse. In early spring, they suffer a period of privation when their winter stores of food are almost exhausted. Although he is a specialist in longevity and the study of old age, he does not know, he says, why they live so long. It would be helpful to decide that they inherit their tendency to long life, but, as Dr. Leaf points out, we do not know of any gene that guarantees long life. There are only genes that predispose one to disease. The Hunzas are probably descended from Greek soldiers who deserted the armies of Alexander the Great. They do not intermarry with other nations, even those who live fairly near them.

The Hunza diet must be largely responsible for keeping these people in good health most of the time and protecting them from the diseases of civilization which are ravaging Western countries: heart and artery disorders, cancer, digestive diseases, diabetes, alcoholism and many others.

23

The Hunzas eat almost no meat or poultry. It is impossible to devote much of their rocky land to raising the many cattle, sheep or goats that would be necessary for much meat-eating. Chickens scratch up and eat seed. Seeds are precious in this remote land, so almost no poultry or eggs are available.

They do have milk, cheese and other dairy products from the few milch animals they keep. Butter is preserved by making it into *ghee.* Cream is boiled to separate the protein part from the fat and the melted fat is *ghee,* which keeps longer than cream keeps. The Hunzas have cheese and cottage cheese, from cow, goat or yak milk, depending on the locality. Butter, milk and yogurt are widely used. Since there is no refrigeration, milk must be soured to keep it for more than a day or two.

John Tobe reports that Hunza cheese is made by pouring milk into a well-tanned goatskin which has been tightly sewed to form a vessel. It is "churned" by simply shaking it up and down until the cream solidifies. Then it is made into a ball, packed in birchbark, placed underneath a water channel and left there for months, or perhaps for years. Tobe reports that it is delicious.

Vegetables, fruits and walnuts are part of the Hunza diet. They garden organically and have for all the years of their existence. No chemicals of any kind are available, or indeed, desired. Every scrap of organic material is carefully saved and composted to be added to the soil in the terraced gardens. Animal manure and human waste are also used. They are carefully composted to destroy any pathogenic bacteria.

The Hunzas cherish their soil. Their lives are spent cultivating it, enriching it, repairing the terraces on which their gardens grow, and irrigating, for there is little rain. Water is brought in from the glaciers high in the rocky cliffs. An ancient, ingenious system of irrigation, all hand-made, performs this formidable job.

Vegetables in the Hunza diet are salad greens, carrots, peas, turnips, squash, potatoes, tomatoes, onions, garlic, beans and pulses like lentils.

The fruit for which Hunza is best known is the apricot, which is an excellent source of the B vitamins, with 2,700 units of vitamin A in every handful. Travellers to that country are impressed with the enormous regard the Hunzakuts have for their apricot trees and the important part this fruit plays in their diet. Hunza apricot trees live for perhaps 100 years. John Tobe says he thinks the reason is that they are grown mostly from seed rather than being grafted. More than 20 varieties of apricots are grown. The Hunzas eat them ripe and fresh from the trees, which most Americans can seldom do, since apricots available in our stores have been picked green so that they will keep until they are shipped to market.

Some apricots are dried by the Hunzas for winter use. The stones are removed and stored. The kernel which is inside the stone is used for apricot oil which is the chief source of fat in the Hunza diet. The job of getting the oil out of the kernel is difficult. The housewife pounds the kernel into mush and rolls it into a fine meal using a stone roller. She adds a little water, then heats the mass over a low fire, kneading it all the time. The oil begins to run out and the cook keeps kneading until the last drop is extracted. The oil is then stored in jars. But usually only a little is made at one time. When this is used, the whole long process must be repeated.

The oil is used for cooking and salad dressings and as a cosmetic and hair dressing. This genuine cold-pressed oil and the fact that it is always used fresh-pressed seem to some observers to be one reason for the good health of the

25

Hunzas. It is a wholesome source of vegetable fat in their diets.

Oil from apricot kernels contains a toxic substance, prussic acid, which is also present in a number of other foods. Primitive people learned long ago that, to make such foods wholesome, they must heat them to drive off the toxic substance. That is undoubtedly one reason for heating the kernel mash as they press out the oil.

Other fruits grown in Hunza are: cherries, apples, peaches, mulberries, grapes and watermelons. The grapes are made into wine without the addition of any sugar. It is fermented for 90 days and is apparently quite potent. The average Hunzakut drinks it only occasionally.

Because Hunza is high in the mountains, wood (the only fuel) is scarce and every scrap of it must be used to best advantage. So generally fruits and vegetables are eaten raw. On the rare occasions when meat is eaten, it is boiled into a stew with vegetables. The only food which must be cooked is bread. And bread is the staple food of the Hunza people, fresh bread baked every day or, for the traveller, every meal. Hunza men carry a bag of wheat with them when they travel. When they stop for meals, they grind it, make up *chapatis* (the kind of bread they eat) and cook them over a tiny fire shielded with three stones.

There is no question whether the bread is wholegrain. There is no way to make it anything else. The entire wheat berry is ground, the flour mixed with a little water, then the dough is kneaded to just the right consistency, flattened into a thin pancake shape and baked on a piece of metal over a small fire. Fresh every day or every meal, *chapatis* may be made of any grain. The Hunzas raise wheat, buckwheat, millet and barley. And often other foods such as lentils, peas or beans are ground into the flour, resulting in a more nourishing bread. For the protein of the legumes comple-

26

ments that of the cereal so that the diner gets the full benefit of all the protein in both foods. This is important in planning a successful vegetarian diet.

There is no indication that the Hunza people would be any less healthy if more meat, eggs and poultry were available. The geography of their country makes it impossible to devote much land to pasture, so they raise only a few animals from which they get milk. Poultry and eggs cannot make up a large part of meals in a land where seeds are valuable and space at a premium.

Two attributes of Hunza life seem to contribute most to good health: their food and the rugged life they lead. First, food is completely natural, raised with dedicated concern for making every inch of soil as rich in nutrients as possible. These nutrients are then absorbed into the food grown there. The irrigation water brought from the glaciers is so rich in minerals that it looks cloudy. It is the only water available for drinking as well as for irrigation.

Second, Hunza life must of necessity involve long hours of extremely vigorous physical labor. All men, women, children and old people must participate. There are almost no tools or farming equipment. Until quite recently, such a heavy job as digging was done using the horns of animals. Now spades and pickaxes are available. There are no wheeled vehicles. Everything must be carried by hand up and down precipitous hillsides. Food must be sown, cultivated, harvested by hand, then prepared, fresh, for every meal by such laborious methods as I have described for making oil, flour and *chapatis*.

There seems to be very good medical evidence that such a vigorous life is the best life if you would be healthy. The Hunza diet, which we could call austere, consists generally of some 1,923 calories compared to the 2,500 calories recommended for the American adult who gets almost no exercise beyond walking to his car and getting in. So, understandably, overweight and obesity are not problems in Hunza.

Music is an important part of Hunza life—a country where crime and juvenile delinquency are unknown. A ball game may involve a group of youngsters pitted against a group of elders who might all be over 70. Neighbors help one another with chores. Children grow up accustomed to hard but rewarding work. Almost no discipline is necessary.

Senator Charles Percy points out in a letter to *Nutrition Today,* "During our visit (to Hunza) I was impressed by the fact that all the residents I spoke with seemed to feel satisfied with their lives—each one felt a sense of accomplishment about his daily work and each felt he or she was still making a contribution to the society. I cannot help but think that psychological well-being is as important to long life as any purely physical factors. . . . As I observed the elderly in Hunza and heard them discuss their work and families with pride, I wished that our own elderly population could live in such a climate of hope."

Because there is no electricity in Hunza and it would be wasteful to use apricot oil for lighting, everyone goes to bed at dusk and gets up at dawn, which is the natural way all diurnal animals arrange their lives. A mounting body of evidence seems to show that getting only natural daylight with no extended time spent under artificial light may also be conducive to good health and longevity. At any rate, the Hunzas are still going strong in their remote, primitive country, still happy and well-satisfied, with no alphabet, no

Footnote: Three months after this chapter was written, I read the account of a reporter, Leo Clancy, who visited Hunza and found that a road has been constructed linking Hunza with the rest of the world. Buses and jeeps bring tourists. An airline company is constructing a modern hotel to house them. Tooth decay, tuberculosis and other infec-

crime, no transportation problems, no energy crisis, no pollution, no sudden shortages of anything, no technology and almost no diseases of civilization.

The gerontologist, Dr. Leaf, visited other nations where remarkable longevity is nothing out of the ordinary. More centenarians live in the Caucasus area known as Abkhazia than in any other locality of the world. This is part of the Georgian Republic of the U.S.S.R., but the population includes Russians, Georgians, Jews, Armenians and Turks. So, says Dr. Leaf, "Genetic inbreeding is not a convincing explanation of the astonishing local record of longevity." Yet all the old people he talked to boasted of relatives who were as old as they.

There are more very old people in the highlands than in the lowlands of this region, according to Dr. Leaf. The incidence of hardening of the arteries among them is half that of other Russian citizens. According to the 1970 census, there are from 4,500 to 5,000 people over the age of 100 in this region. Since there are only 5,000,000 people in the Georgian Republic of the U.S.S.R., this means that of every 100,000 Georgians, 39 are 100 years old or more—13 times more than there are in every 100,000 Americans. In Azerbaijan there are 21 times·more.

Georgians eat everything available—meat, dairy products, an abundance of vegetables and fruits. Many of the oldsters also drink and smoke. Like every tourist who visits Georgia, Dr. Leaf was overwhelmed by Georgian hospitality. "Within minutes," he says, "the women would have a table buried under its load of bread, *mamaligia* (a kind of corn-

tious diseases are ravaging the people who have also become greedy and jealous. The Mir, ruler of Hunza, says sadly, "Modern technology is to blame for many of our troubles." The New York Times, April 21, 1974, announced all-inclusive three week tours to Hunza for any tourist who has the necessary three thousand dollars.

meal mush), cucumbers, onions, tomatoes, garlic, cheese, roasted and boiled chicken, sauce and spices, boiled mutton, goat's meat and beef. Fresh fruits and sometimes a rich pastry or a platter of chocolate candies completed the setting."

Early toasts were drunk with homemade vodka or a local brandy. Then the serious toasting began, using Georgian wine, which is a quite famous beverage among gourmets. And, says Dr. Leaf, the old people joined in all the toasts, ate and drank as heartily as the younger ones.

It is well to remember that Georgia is an extremely isolated part of the U.S.S.R. and that, up until quite recently, such things as chocolate candy were unknown. The traditional Georgian "candy" is *chuchkella*. In *Russian Cooking*, the Papashvilys describe it.

"Making *chuchkella* called for time and patience. Perfect, unbroken walnut halves were strung on a heavy thread that was knotted at one end and tied in a loop at the other. These strings were dipped into the juice of sweet grapes that had been boiled and slightly thickened with flour. They were next hung to dry, then re-dipped and re-dried until the *chuchkella* was about an inch thick. In the autumn every balcony and arbor was trimmed with rows of drying tapers, their fruity sweetness filling the air and attracting swarms of tipsy bees and expectant children. Finally the *chuchkella* were sliced, each piece transformed into a perfect intaglio of convoluted ivory set in a circlet of glowing jasper."

George Papashvily, who grew up in Georgia some 70 years ago, tells us that his people have lived in that same sweet mountainous country ("most like paradise") for 7,000 years. They have lived for most of these years on bountiful fare: wheat and corn, fish, game, beans, wild onions and asparagus, young nettles, mallow, sorrel, sarsaparilla and a favorite salad dish called *donduri* in Georgian, which is purslane cooked and prepared with a dressing of oil, lemon juice, garlic and salt. Of herbs they use tarragon, coriander, dill, basil, oregano, thyme, savory, mint, marigolds and fenugreek.

For fruits they have cherries, pears, apples, quinces, figs, grapes, pomegranates, filberts, chestnuts, Persian walnuts. Walnuts were pounded into paste for many cookery uses. Georgians made—and still make—sauces of tomatoes, garlic, barberries, aloeberries, green grapes, pomegranates.

The Georgian yogurt is called *matsoni*. You make it of buffalo milk or cow's milk. Says George, "A quart of whole milk (that of the water buffalo, very rich and sweet works better) is brought to a rolling boil and poured into a crock or wide-mouthed jar. Then when the milk cools to luke-warm, a half cup of 'starter' from a previous batch is stirred into it with a wooden spoon; (the temperature of the milk is important, for the culture is a living thing and likes a pleasant climate). The vessel is covered and put into a warm place where it rests undisturbed for three or four hours until it thickens. It may then be refrigerated." Says Papashvily, "Georgians eat few sweets for dessert. Our dessert was fruit."

Sula Benet, Professor of Anthropology at Hunter College in New York, writing about the Abkhasians (U.S.S.R.) in *Family Health,* December, 1972, and *The New York Times,* December 26, 1971, tells us these folks have been there for at least 1,000 years. There are 100,000 of them. Dr. Benet says it is as if all the physical and mental changes which we associate with aging had stopped at a certain point. Most of the elderly Abkhasians work regularly. They have good eyesight and, mostly, their own teeth. They may walk two or three miles a day and swim in their mountain streams. With good posture right into old age, they are handsome and healthy.

They have no words meaning "old people." Those over

31

100 are called "long living people." According to most recent official statistics, 2.57 percent of all their people are over 90. In the U.S.A. the figure is something like .4 percent. There were no reported cases of mental illness or cancer in a nine year study of 123 people all over 100 years old.

An Abkhasian is never "retired." He does whatever work he is capable of doing and thinks this is an eminently satisfactory way of living, for his status increases as he ages. Men and women over 100 work an average four-hour day on the collective farm. Overeating is considered dangerous. Fat people are regarded as ill. An Abkhasian cannot get fat, they say, for what a ridiculous figure he would be on horseback!

At all three daily meals Abkhasians eat *abista,* a cornmeal mash cooked in water without salt. This is their bread. They eat it warm with pieces of goat cheese inside. Meat is eaten several times a week. Most people drink two glasses of buttermilk a day. When they eat eggs, which is infrequently, they boil or fry them with cheese. Other foods are fresh fruits, grapes, fresh vegetables, including green onions, tomatoes, cucumbers, cabbage, pickled vegetables and lima beans "cooked slowly for hours, mashed and flavored with a sauce of onions, peppers, garlic, pomegranate juice and pepper."

The peppery sauce is served in a separate dish for anyone to use. And there is always plenty of garlic available. They drink neither coffee nor tea, but use a local red wine, in small quantities. They do not use sugar, but have some honey. Toothaches are rare. The Abkhasians' caloric intake is 23 percent lower than that of industrial workers in their area and contains twice the amount of vitamin C.

Many Soviet health authorities believe it is the buttermilk and pickled vegetables that account for the Abkhasians' fabled longevity. These foods help to destroy harmful bacteria in the intestine, they say, and prevent the development of hardening of the arteries.

Dr. Sam Rosen, who reported on the health of the African Mabaans, found that the Abkhasians have remarkable hearing powers which he thought was due to their diet being low in saturated fats and including many fruits and vegetables. All foods, including meat and poultry, are cooked for a minimum of time. Anything that can be eaten raw is eaten raw. Nuts are pounded into butter and used for cooking.

Dr. Benet tells the story of a young couple who moved into the city, Sukhumi, bringing the husband's elderly mother with them. They hired a maid who did all the housework. The mother began to fail and complained that she was dying. A doctor, hastily summoned, said that she must be taken back to her village. "Inactivity will kill her," he said. Back home, working a full schedule, she revived at once, and is still there, happily being useful.

Shirali Mislimov, an Azerbaijan whom the Soviet government authorities say is 168 years old, was described by Lloyd Shearer in *Parade* for September 24, 1972. He works in his orchard, eats sparingly, mostly vegetables and fruits, drinks wine and rarely worries. Mislimov wrote recently to a California gerontologist, "I get up early in the morning, work in my garden, go to bed just after ten in the evening, never sleep in the daytime and take daily walks of nearly one kilometer (one-half mile)." Shearer refers to Mislimov as "a personage of serenity, peace of mind and an apparently endless will to live."

Dr. Benet thinks that the culture of these primitive people may have a lot to do with their longevity. She recommends the high degree of integration in their lives and their sense of group identity. They have, she says, a

33

feeling of personal security and continuity. Their small world has changed very little over all these years. And they are able, somehow, to adapt themselves to some of the conditions brought by outside society, yet maintain their own culture.

Chapter
4

The North American Indians, before and after Their "Discovery"

The Indians we learned most about in school were those who lived in the area that is now New England and who taught the early colonists how to survive in a country where almost nothing was like it had been in England. The Indians taught our forefathers how to "cull out the finest seede, to observe the fittest season, to keep distance for holes and measure for hills, to worme it and weed it; to prune it and dress it, as occasion shall require," according to a contemporary observer, who also tells us that the Indians were so industrious they would not allow a weed "to advance his audacious head above their infant corn, or an undermining worme to spoile his spurnes."

Each Indian family had its own garden, or several. Sometimes they were a mile apart and when work in one garden was over the family might move its shelter over to another field. They planted with sharpened digging sticks. The hills of corn were three feet apart, not in straight rows. Into each hill went two or three fish, four kernels of corn, four of beans, squash and pumpkins. Hoes made of seashells or wood were used to heap up dirt over the hills.

The Indians grew several varieties of corn—red, blue, yellow and white. They planted white, black, red, yellow

35

and blue beans. The corn stalks supported the beans, which were all climbing varieties. The squash and pumpkins flourished on the ground among the corn stalks.

Indian women harvested the corn, dried it and stored it in trenches in the ground in large grass sacks. In 1935, Dr. Charles C. Willoughby, author of *Antiquities of the New England Indians,* found 35 such cache holes in an area of less than half an acre in the Kennebec River Valley.

The pattern of eating went like this among the Indians in old New England. Roasting ears and other garden produce until frost. Then fresh game until the snow became too deep. In winter, meals consisted of dried corn and beans, acorns, nuts, dried berries, dried meat and fish and whatever fresh game, fish and clams could be found. Spring brought plenty of fish, as well as ducks and geese on their migratory trails.

Dr. Willoughby states that the amount of corn stored for winter consumption by an Indian community might be assessed from the fact that the Pilgrims in 1622, short of provisions, obtained from the Indians on Cape Cod 26 to 28 hogsheads of corn and beans.

Many traditional New England dishes are derived from Indian recipes. The Pilgrims learned about clambakes from the Indians. A deep pit was lined with flat stones on which a fire was built. When the stones were white-hot, the embers were removed and a layer of seaweed was laid down. Clams and roasting ears alternated on top of the seaweed. The final "bake" was covered with seaweed and a blanket of wet hide to keep everything moist.

Succotash was an Indian dish arrived at by combining whatever was at hand in the way of corn and beans with other foods added as desired. The word "succotash" is from an Indian word meaning "husked corn." Hominy is dried corn ground into meal and cooked with water into mush. This name, too, is derived from an Indian word. Corn pone is unleavened corn bread, flat, cooked on a griddle or in the embers of a fire.

Almost anything could go into the cornmeal mush which the English settlers called "frumenty." An Indian woman or an English housewife might toss into the bubbling mush shad, eels, alewives or herring, dried or fresh, some meat in pieces, roots, squash, acorns, chestnuts or walnuts. The Indians removed the bitterness from acorns by boiling them in lye made from rotten maplewood ashes. Hickory nuts were crushed, shell and all, and mixed with water. The oil which rose to the top was skimmed off and saved. Motherless babies were sometimes fed a boiled mixture of crushed black walnuts and a little water, mixed with some finely-ground cornmeal. Groundnuts (*Apios tuberosa*) were a staple food. This is a climbing perennial which bears tubers on its roots which are about the size of eggs. Groundnuts were eaten by the Pilgrims during the hungry winter of 1623.

The Hopi Indians of Arizona were fine gardeners who supported themselves in a dry climate by careful use of water. They raised beans, squash, pumpkins, sunflower seeds and corn, of which they had many varieties. In lean years they supplemented this diet with desert fare: mesquite beans, prickly pears and many wild seeds, roots and berries.

The Crow Indians of the Western plains lived chiefly on buffalo which they boiled in rawhide vessels over a fire. They also dried it in thin strips by the heat of the sun and made it into "pemmican" which is lean meat, pounded fine and mixed with fat, then flavored with berries. This food was a staple of explorers, for it would keep for a long time. In spring the Crows had "cottonwood ice cream," a frothy gelatinous sap from the cottonwood tree, which they obtained by peeling off the outer bark of the tree and scraping the exposed area.

The Iroquois made bread of the bark of maple trees, pond lily roots, wild parsnips and groundnuts. They collected many kinds of nuts every autumn, as well as fruits and berries to dry and store. They had maple sugar and syrup. They ate quail, partridge, wild duck, frogs, turtles and their eggs, crayfish and clams, and birds' eggs. Poor Iroquois also gathered the excrement of deer and made a kind of soup of it. They trapped fish in weirs and nets, and harpooned eels. Before planting their corn or beans, they soaked the seed in herb concoctions or medicines which hastened the germination. They knew how to save seed which appeared to produce superior crops, in the best tradition of agronomists and plant geneticists.

The Haida Indians of British Columbia used a fish called the "candlefish" which was so oily that, when it was dried, it could be used as a candle by inserting a wick. They grew herring spawn on hemlock branches sunk in the sea. They boiled it with herbs and berries and pressed it into cakes or ate it pounded and mixed with water, then beaten to a creamy consistency. Or they enjoyed it in a decomposed condition after it had been buried in boxes on the beach. When the Haida had a party they heaped whatever food had not been eaten onto plates which they sent home with their guests. The clean plates were returned the next day, sometimes with a gift.

The Micmac Indians of Eastern Canada lived mostly on wild game, fish and shellfish. They roasted meat and fish on spits propped before their fires, turning it to cook on all sides. Fat was melted on a grooved stone and ran into a birchbark container. When this container was full, the fat was melted again and put into a seal bladder or stomach which was used for a bag.

Of vegetable foods they ate wild "potatoes" which were in reality wild carrots. They robbed the squirrels' stores of beechnuts, ate huckleberries, blueberries, serviceberries, cran-berries—all of which they dried in the sun and made into cakes for winter storage. They used twigs of yellow birch, winterberries and roots of sassafras for tea, as well as spruce leaves, waxberries, tips of young maple leaves, leaves or bark of hemlock and chips of rock maple.

Maple sap was boiled and made into sugar loaves. When early French settlers finally persuaded the Micmacs that they should eat some bread, they made it out of corn-meal and cooked it in the sand. Live coals were scraped away, the dough was put directly into the hot sand, covered with sand, and left there to bake for an hour or so. As late as 1890 some old people among the Micmacs refused to eat bread unless it had been made in this fashion, we are told.

Dr. Diamond Jenness in *Indians of Canada,* says that the Iroquois planted sunflowers among their squash, beans and corn and used oil from the seeds as ointment. Indians in Virginia made bread and soup of sunflower seeds. The Iroquois determined the site of their villages by the fertility of the land. A contemporary writer tells us that in 1677 the Onondaga with about 350 men in their community, built their village on a hill, cleared the land and planted corn for two miles around. Ten years later, when the French General Frontenac attacked this tribe, it took his men three days to destroy the growing corn.

Wild rice was harvested by Indians around the Great Lakes. In a canoe lined with birchbark, a man sat with a hand on each side. He took hold of the stalks of wild rice, knocked the heads of the plants against the inside of the canoe until he had an entire boat full. One canoe might hold up to 12 bushels. An industrious harvester could fill his canoe three times a day. On scaffolds lined with thick grass, the rice was laid and "gentle" fires were kept going beneath it, while the rice was turned until it was dry. Then it was pounded in a mortar to remove the husks, and stored in bags made of rushes.

Around the Great Lakes wild rice is still harvested in much the same way. This is the reason it is so expensive—getting it takes time, patience and skill, three attributes not very highly esteemed by our modern agricultural establishment.

Indians in British Columbia ate several kinds of seaweed, the camas root (*Quamasia*), elderberries, gooseberries, soapberries (*Sapindus*), huckleberries, currants, crabapples and many other roots and berries, all of them gathered by the women and stored for winter. However, meat and fish are necessities in cold climates, so all the Northern Indians relied heavily on them.

Dr. Jenness tells us that no country in the world offered its earliest people such a wealth of available food as North America. Both oceans teemed with salmon which migrated annually up the rivers. For many years they were so numerous that many fish were pushed high and dry on the banks. There were abundant shellfish in both oceans, as well as halibut and cod. There were seals, whales, sea lions and sea otters on the West Coast. In interior lakes were whitefish, sturgeon, lake trout, salmon trout, pike, pickerel.

Game animals abounded. Bear, deer and rabbits were available everywhere. Moose, woodland caribou and porcupine lived in the eastern forests. Huge herds of antelope and bison roamed the plains. Sheep and goats lived in the Western mountains while elk wandered in the foothills and mountain caribou grazed on the plateaus. Herds of caribou were so immense that no one could estimate their numbers. Ducks, geese, swans, grouse and ptarmigan were plentiful in some seasons.

But not always. And in lean seasons the going was hard. The Indians had to move from one locality to another to follow the movements of the deer or the migrations of waterfowl or salmon. Differing times of the year meant hardship to different nations. A Cree Indian is quoted as begging for a period of gale so that he might hunt deer in deep snow. "I took my rattle and tambour," said he, "and sang to the Great Spirit and the Manito of the Winds; the next morning I did the same, and took out of my medicine bag sweet smelling herbs and laid them on a small fire to the Manito. I smoked and sang to him for a wind, but he shut his ears and would not listen to me; for three days I did the same, but he kept his ears shut. . . ."

Famines and hardships limited population growth. Among those Indians who had no cereals, infants had to be nursed by their mothers up to the age of three, for there was no way to prepare a diet of fish and meat to make it suitable for such little ones. This, of course, also limited the population.

Dr. Jenness reminds us that a migratory outdoor life, with man pitting his wits against the habits and instincts of the game animals, develops close observation powers and a deep perception of the mysteries of nature. The Indians were expert naturalists. They knew the life histories of the birds and animals they needed for food. They knew when and where they migrated, how and what they ate. They knew every stage of the salmon from egg to adult life. One group of Indians on Vancouver Island stocked their streams with salmon eggs, as our fisheries experts do today. Their interest in the environment around them and their willingness to experiment led them to discover the medicinal properties of many plants. Early colonists owe their Indian neighbors a great debt for their help in identifying plants with healing properties.

The California Indians used the following seeds and nuts as food: California Buckeye (*Aesculus californica*) which contained a slightly toxic substance, hence needed leaching, as acorns do. The ground flour was made into soup. According to Muriel Sweet in *Common Edible and Useful Plants of the West,* buckeye flour must be leached by pouring water over it at least ten times to carry off the poisonous material. The best leaching was done by letting the water of a small stream flow over the ground flour for ten days. The flour was then cooked as a pudding.

California Laurel (*Umbellularia californica*), also called California Bay or Peppernut, had seeds which were stored for winter use. The seeds were also parched, cracked and eaten or made into "bread." Screwbeans (*Prosopis pubescens*) were cooked in a pot lined with leaves. The time of cooking varied. Some Indians left them there for days, others for months. Then they were stored for winter.

Chia (*Salvia Columbariae*) was one of the most important sources of vegetable protein food. The seeds are small. Indians harvested them by bending the heads of the plants over a basket and beating the seeds into it with a paddle. Or the entire plant was harvested and the seeds were threshed out with rods on a hard earth surface. The Indians stirred them into water for a beverage. And they made gruel of *chia.* Although it sounds apocryphal, an Indian could supposedly keep marching for 24 hours on one teaspoon of *chia* seed. They baked it into cakes and used it to flavor other kinds of flour.

Tansy-mustard or peppergrass (*Descurania pinnata*) has fine small seeds which were gathered, parched, ground into flour and made into mush. It was also used for poultices. Pinyon (*Pinus monophylla*) is the one-leaved pine which provided much high-protein food in its seeds which were hidden in the cones. The cones were gathered and set on fire to burn off the pitch, then the seeds easily separated from the cones. They were parched and eaten, as they still are in

42

many parts of California.

Jojoba or Goatnut (*Simmondsia chinensis*) has large seeds rich in oil which were eaten without any further preparation. Dr. Edward K. Balls in *Early Uses of California Plants,* tells us that at one time these nuts were sold in Los Angeles drug stores as hair restorers. They were boiled and the oil was rubbed into the hair. Unfortunately we can provide no photographs that will testify to the results. Mexicans made a beverage of these nuts—roasted them, then ground them and mixed them with the yolk of a hardboiled egg, adding a vanilla bean, then boiled the whole mixture with water, milk and sugar. Early white settlers learned to make the beverage, too.

Muriel Sweet mentions that the soft center of the cone of the Digger Pine (*Pinus Sabiniana*) was roasted for about 20 minutes in hot ashes and yielded a syrupy food which the Indians liked. The seed was usually eaten raw.

Here are some uses the California Indians made of the berries or fruit of native flora. There seems to have been plenty to eat at any season of the year. California Fan Palm (*Washingtonia filifera*) carries large clusters of berries which turn black when they are ripe. The Indians gathered them, roasted them, ate them whole or ground them into flour for cakes. Wild grapes (*Vitis californica*) were used as we use them today, for eating, beverages, wine, jellies, preserves. Barberry and Mountain Grape (*Berberis*) berries were used as flavoring in soup or for wine or jelly.

California wild rose (*Rosa californica*) has fruit, which are called rose hips, well-known these days for their fantastic vitamin C content, as well as their vitamin A. The Indians used them for tea or ate the hips right from the bush. Chokecherry (*Prunus demissa*) has bright red berries whose name suggests their acrid taste. The Indians leached out the acid by pouring water through them, then ground them and ate

43

the boiled, dried pulp. They also make fine wine or jelly.

Western serviceberry (*Amelanchier pallida*) has purplish to black seeds which the Indians dried for winter use. They also made them into a cake. They would break off a bit of cake to flavor a soup. They also used the berries to make *pemmican,* the convenience food for travellers. Blackberries, thimbleberries (*Rubus parviflora*), Christmasberries (*Heteromeles arbutifolia*), scarlet sumac, were all used by California Indians.

Manzanita (*Arctostaphylos*) berries formed a basic food for the Indians. They gathered the red berries, ate them raw or cooked, or ground them into meal for porridge. Sometimes they made cider from them. Blueberry elder (*Sambucus caerulea*) had berries which the Indians dried in the sun and put away for winter use. Later, white residents of California used them with sugar for pies, muffins or pancakes.

Tuna or Indian fig (*Opuntia Ficus-indica*) is a cactus. The Indians ate the fruit, after peeling it to remove the spines. A syrup was made by boiling tuna and straining out the seeds. Spanish settlers boiled it even longer and made an almost black paste which they called *Quesa de Tuna.* Toyon (*Heteromeles arbutifolia*), also known as California holly or Christmasberry, was the source of cider and berries for the eating, but first the bunches were held over a fire or tossed in a basket with hot pebbles to take away some of the bitterness.

California Indians used the leaves, flowers, stalks and roots of the following plants.

Most important was an *agave,* two varieties of which, *A. deserti* and *A. utahensis,* were referred to by the Indians as *mescal,* a word which we use today for an alcoholic beverage they drink in Mexico. In spring, when the agave buds were beginning to show, Indians came from miles

44

around and camped for weeks at places where there was plenty of agave growing. They cut the crisp "cabbages," which were the buds, collected and cooked them in a communal oven. A ditch was dug and a hot fire built. Then the ashes were raked out and a layer of agave leaves or grass was laid down. The cabbage-like heads were laid on the hot leaves and covered with another layer of leaves and grass, or grass and sand. The oven was left to bake until the next day. The charred leaves were removed from the baked heads, revealing brown juicy centers, very sweet and nourishing. Some of these were eaten on the spot, the rest were made into cakes, dried and stored for winter. They could be eaten dry or slipped into a soup.

Mesquite (*Prosopis juliflora*) produces long yellow beans which the Indians stored, dry, in coarse open-work basket "granaries." They were ground and made into meal which was mixed with water and left to stand and ferment for a few hours. Large quantities of the fresh beans were also eaten raw. The pulp of these beans is a sweet and nutritious food, according to Dr. Balls. It was made into a beverage wherever the plants grew. One tribe of Indians found that mixing some soil with the ground meal improved its taste.

Mariposa lily or sego lily (*Calochortus Nuttallii*) grows from a bulb which was gathered in great quantities by the Indians, using a digging stick. They cooked the bulbs in rock-lined earth ovens. Camas or Quamash (*Camassia Quamash*) is another plant with a bulbous root which was the most important bulb food of the Indians. The bulbs were baked in the "oven" and emerged soft, dark brown and nutritious, tasting a little like chestnuts. They were eaten or made into cakes to be stored.

Tule potato (*Sagittaria latifolia*), the common arrowhead, also grew from a bulb which the Indians cherished.

45

Indian women, wading in the water where the plant grew, and pushing small canoes before them, loosened the tubers with their feet so they floated to the surface of the water. The bulbs were skinned and eaten.

Cat-tail (*Typha latifolia*) provides bread made from its pollen. Now we know that pollen has a high protein content. This must have been a most nutritious bread. The root was roasted and consumed. The young shoots were gathered and eaten like asparagus. Beavertail (*Opuntia basilaris*) was valued for its fruit which was gathered, cleaned of spines and cooked for about 12 hours. The immature fruits of the plant, the flower buds and the joints were also eaten.

Bracken fern (*Pteridium aquilinum*) was used when the tops were very young and tender. Pioneers in the West soaked the tops in water for 24 hours, then cooked them like vegetables. In New Brunswick and Nova Scotia, fern "fiddleheads" are still considered a delicacy. They are the tender green shoots of ferns which are cooked like asparagus and taste even better.

Watercress (*Nasturtium officinale*) was used by the Indians and early settlers mostly as a medicinal plant. Probably its large content of vitamin A and vitamin C performed the magic. Indian pond lilies (*Nuphar polysepalum*) were valuable for the .rootstock, which was baked, and for their seeds which were made into bread and soup. Dr. Balls lists these plants, parts of which were made into beverages by the California Indians: Manzanita, Mexican tea or squaw tea (*Ephedra*), barberry (*Mahonia*), barrel cactus (*Echinocactus acanthodes*), sugar bush (*Rhus integrifolia*).

The diet of the California Indians must have been much more varied and plentiful than that of other American Indians. The supply of wild food was more than enough, practically the year around. Indians drew their food from

46

hillsides and canyons which white settlers and later residents consider barren locations. If the supply of one food failed, in California, there were other foods available. If the buffalo unaccountably shifted, or the salmon failed to run, the very existence of peoples in other regions was shaken to its foundation. But in California the wide distribution of available foods prevented a failure of a single crop from producing starvation.

A gathering society gathers insects and small animals as easily as berries and nuts. The California Indians ate grasshoppers, caterpillars, maggots, snails, shellfish, crayfish, turtles, minnows, gophers, lizards and small birds. All these added considerably to the essential protein of their diets.

In *Nutrition and Physical Degeneration* Dr. Price tells us that he found, among the British Columbia Indians, a plant which was used to treat diabetes. A patient brought in for an operation was found to have diabetes. Telling the story of his condition, the Indian revealed that he controlled it by taking a hot water infusion of the root of a plant called devil's club. Our horticultural encyclopedia lists the botanical name of this shrub as *Oplopanax horridum.* Presumably "horridum" because of its thorns. It is a native of the West coast from Alaska to California, and belongs to the Aralia family to which ginseng also belongs. It is sometimes called *Fatsia horrida.*

Medical researchers should certainly investigate this plant. It may contain some trace mineral in abundance which helps to regulate blood sugar. Two isolated incidents have been reported in medical journals in which alfalfa tea was used to regulate the wild swings of blood sugar in an uncontrolled diabetic who would not control his disorder with diet. Doctors theorized that it may have been the alfalfa's large content of the trace mineral manganese which wrought this seeming miracle.

47

Dr. Price points out that animal skeletons are rarely found in areas where large game animals made up much of the diet of the Northern Indians. Skeletal remains that are found are piles of finely-broken bone chips or splinters that have been cracked to obtain as much as possible of the marrow and minerals of the bones. These Indians obtained much of their quota of vitamin A and vitamin D from the organs of the animals they ate. Children, especially, were given bone marrow as a substitute for milk.

Dr. Price relates the story of two prospectors, both doctors of science and engineering, who lost their way in the Far North and made a forced march, abandoning all their elaborate and expensive equipment. One day one of the men suffered an agonizing pain in his eyes. It was not snow blindness for the men had dark glasses to protect their eyes from the glare. A passing Indian caught a fish from a nearby stream and indicated that the prospector should eat the flesh of the head and the flesh back of the eyes, including the eyes. Within a few days the pain subsided and in two more days his eyes were nearly normal. The prospector told Dr. Price he had been suffering from *xerophthalmia,* caused by lack of vitamin A. Eye tissues, especially the retina, are rich in this vitamin. In many primitive countries animal eye tissues are a favored and very great delicacy, possibly because of their relation to eye health.

Comparing the native diet of the Indians of the Far North with that of the white man, Dr. Price found that the Indian diet provided 5.8 times more calcium, 5.8 times more phosphorus, 2.7 times more iron, 4.3 times more magnesium, 15 times more copper, 8.8 times more iodine and at least ten times more of the fat soluble vitamins.

Life expectancy for American Indians today is 64 years, significantly below the 71-year span for white Americans. The leading causes of death from disease vary greatly from those of white Americans. Indians die from diseases of the heart at the rate of 180.9 deaths per 100,000 compared to 57.2 per 100,000 for white Americans. Influenza and pneumonia claim twice as many Indians, as do diseases of early infancy. Cirrhosis of the liver kills 39 Indians in every 100,000, compared to only 14 whites. Diabetes mellitus is about the same in the two groups. Tuberculosis claims five times more Indians than whites. And digestive diseases of many kinds (colitis, gastroenteritis, etc.) kill almost five times more Indians than whites. Indians have five times as many cases of gonorrhea, eight times as many cases of hepatitis, 10 times as many cases of strep throat, 20 times as many of meningitis and 100 times as many cases of dysentery as the rest of our population.

Indians are today considered the most disadvantaged people in the United States. Two thirds of them have no running water in their homes but haul drinking water from potentially contaminated sources. Most live in poorly heated, overcrowded homes.

The Public Health Service offers the explanation that the Indians live under primitive sanitary conditions. It is abundantly obvious that malnutrition is also closely involved with all these disorders. Before the coming of the white man Indians were free from these plagues. Their water and air were pure, their food wholesome, their way of life, established over many thousands of years, guaranteed them enough nourishment for healthy lives and an environment that would continue to provide nourishment as well as housing and clothing. These are things which our present Department of Agriculture and World Health Organization cannot guarantee for more than a short time into the future.

Today, beset by overwhelming poverty, forced to conform to the regulations of an industrial society which makes no effort to understand their needs, and a government which has broken every treaty our forefathers made with the Indians, they represent the most heinous reproach to the conscience of America.

The Primitive People of South America

When the Spanish explorers and conquerors came to South America, they found an advanced agricultural civilization and a well organized economic system. Indians whose ancestors had lived here for thousands of years had already discovered the uses of hundreds of plants and animals. They cultivated plants from which they made food, flavorings, drugs, poisons, fibers, clothing, gums, dyes and paints. The world owes to them at least 40 important foods which have improved life for people in other parts of the world.

Frederick Peterson in his book *Ancient Mexico,* tells us that the Indians of South America cultivated more than 50 species of beans, including lima beans, green or "snap" beans and kidney beans. They ate them with chili peppers which ranged from delicate, sweet morsels to peppers so "hot" they seemed to fill one's mouth with hot coals. They raised pumpkins, squash and calabash (gourds) for more than 2,000 years before Columbus.

Indians in Mexico and South America grew potatoes, yams (*Dioscorea*), sweet potatoes, which come from the morning glory family (*Ipomoea batatas*), and arrowroot (*Maranta arundinacea*). Peanuts were a staple food. Popcorn, which Indians called parched corn, was used by travellers, since it was easy to heat and pop open over a fire. And the Indians strung it into chains for decoration, as we do on our Christmas trees. Chewing gum comes from a Mexican tree, the *Sapodilla* (*Sapota achras*). It gives a sticky milky sap which is the base of chicle used for chewing gum. The ancient Mexicans used it to clean their teeth. What a mockery of this fine healthful product is our American chewing gum which, well-sugared as it is, destroys teeth as viciously as any other sticky sweet!

The breadnut tree (*Brosimum alicastrum*) yields a nut which the Mexicans roasted and ate like potatoes or ground into flour and made into bread. Several kinds of onions were grown and often eaten with *xictomatl*. This Aztec name was later corrupted into "tomato" when this vitamin C-rich food was taken to Europe.

The Aztecs also smoked tobacco. A Spanish traveller in the 1580's put it this way, "And they have some tubes or reeds, which are full of tobacco called *picietl* which is ground up with lime and other roots and liquidambar and they make from these ingredients a mass with which they fill their smoke tubes that they call *poquietl,* and burning the point of this tube they stick the other end in their mouth and suck on it, and draw out a smoke that does not smell bad. And then they blow smoke, dispatching it from the mouth, and it is so strong that it makes one sleepy." And, in our time, cancerous as well.

"Food made from poison" is what E. Hyatt Verrill calls *manioc* in his book *Foods America Gave the World.* This was a staple food maintaining many cultures and nations in South America. Its origins are lost in time. There is not even a fable giving any hint of its source. Centuries before Columbus arrived, this food had spread through the American tropics, South and Central America and the West Indies. In most places it was an important food and in many places it was the most important root food.

Manioc is also called *yuca, cassava, mandioca, casbi, casabi, manihot* and *rumu* in different parts of the world. The enormous roots of this tropical plant may yield as much as 13 tons per acre of a fleshy, starchy food. The botanical name is *Manihot*. The sweet variety is known as *Manihot dulcis Aipi* and the bitter variety *Manihot esculenta*. Verrill tells us that *manioc* may have been first cultivated by the pre-Incans of Peru or by Indians who lived in the West Indies, by the Aztec or Mayan people or by the Carib tribes of northern South America.

In any case, there are two varieties, one tasting bitter, the other sweet. People in various localities prefer one or the other, depending mostly on what their ancestors ate. Both are poisonous in the raw state. Verrill understandably marvels at how the Indians discovered ways of processing these roots to make them edible. Obviously it could not have been done by experimentation, for anyone eating the unsuccessful experiments would have died. Probably these ancient peoples discovered quite by accident that certain processes would take out the prussic acid and render both varieties of manioc perfectly safe to eat. Modern chemists know that prussic acid is easily driven off by heat, but the ancient Indians were not chemists.

And, as Verrill points out, even our best chemists have not devised any better method of processing *manioc* than the Indians devised. It is to them, rather than to our rich modern food technology establishment, that we owe the food which now comes packed in supermarket cartons under the name of tapioca. Tapioca is made of *manioc*.

Much of the poison is just under the skin, so South American women peel the roots carefully, then grate them. They did this in olden times by chopping or grinding the roots between stones, or they used a rough grater made of

53

wood with sharp chips of quartz and other hard stones set in it.

The mass of pulverized *manioc* was then put in a cylinder-shaped basket which could be compressed by pressing the ends together. It was called a *metapee.* This hung on a tree in such a way that the weight of one or two women would compress the basket, pressing out the toxic juice. The pulp which remained was put through a sieve, then baked on hot stones or on a sheet of iron. This baking drove off the last of the poison. When made into flat cakes and baked, *manioc* will keep almost indefinitely.

The poisonous juice is boiled down into a thick syrup (also harmless) called *cassareep,* which used to be the basis for Worcestershire sauce. At present soy sauce is used instead. *Cassareep* can preserve meat, says Verrill. Every Indian family in Guiana has its jar of this syrupy stuff which never spoils. Meat is added, the tougher the better, and comes out with a most unusual and delicious flavor. More sauce is added to the jar from time to time, as more *manioc* is processed.

South American Indians make an alcoholic beverage of the dried meal left after the *manioc* has been sieved. To get fast fermentation the women chew the meal and spit it out into troughs where the enzymes from the saliva bring about fermentation. The women are selected for their perfect teeth and they go through an elaborate ritual of cleansing and rinsing their mouths before they begin to chew the *manioc.* Verrill reports that the final drink is a ceremonial beverage which, when he was in South America, it was mandatory to drink if you would not insult your South American host. It tastes not unlike hard cider. The Arawak Indians had 24 varieties of *manioc,* along with five varieties of corn, potatoes and beans.

Carleton Beals in *Nomads and Empire Builders,* tells us

that in Tierra del Fuego (those islands at the very tip of South America) the "canoe people" hunted and ate leopard, crab and monk seals, sea lions, sea elephants, turtles, whales, fish, all manner of crustaceans, including barnacles, sea spiders and sea urchins. They also ate deer, rodents and *guanaco,* a camel-like animal which lived by grazing on peat moss.

In Southern Chile there are raspberries, gooseberries and Chilean lilies (which are like our cucumbers.) The inhabitants eat *mara* (a rodent like our rabbit), rats, foxes, a sort of gopher, the *rhea* (an ostrich-like bird), geese, hawks, penguins and birds' eggs. In some places, Beals says, fish are so plentiful they can be scooped up by hand.

The Amazon valley contains the most varied plant life anywhere on the planet, according to Beals, and the Indians who live there make use of an astonishing number of plants. The Xingu tribe transplanted the wild *piqui* trees close to their dwellings so that they might use their edible nuts which were 95 percent oil. Other tribes tied together the stems of wild grasses so that their seeds would fall into small heaps that could more easily be gathered. And they made a salt substitute of certain fibers and fruits which were processed into a brown or gray powder.

The Macundu people extracted the oil from the bark of the *Maquema* tree to treat dysentery and used the leaves of an aromatic myrtle to clean their teeth and treat bad breath. From very ancient times the people knew many herb cures, drugs, aphrodisiacs and abortives, as well as pesticides, poisons, antidotes for poisons and for various bites and stings.

There are cashew nuts and Brazil nuts which were sometimes cooked with *manioc* or ground corn. The Chachapayas tree (*caryocar amygdaliferum*) grows a spiny chestnut which is soft and buttery with lots of oil in it.

In *Everyday Life of the Aztecs,* Warwick Bray tells us

that meat was a luxury for the average family in Aztec times. The housewife spent some six hours every day preparing corn which was the basis for all meals. The kernels were steeped in lime overnight to loosen the hulls, the kernels were boiled and skinned. Then they were ground to powder by crushing them between a grooved stone roller and a *metate* (a stone slab standing on three little legs.) The corn was then usually made into *tortillas,* which are unleavened pancakes cooked on flat clay griddles. They are dry and tasteless after a few hours, so they were made fresh for every meal!

An Aztec child might have half a tortilla as a daily ration, along with other food like fruits and vegetables. By the time he was five years old, he might have a whole tortilla and by the age of 13 he might eat two a day. This is not a diet that produces obesity in children, especially since these very active little ones had many chores that had to be performed every day. The lime used to soak the corn kernels provided the calcium which the children needed and which was almost lacking in the corn.

How did it happen that the Aztecs did not get pellagra? This deficiency disease decimated areas of our own South not so many years ago when corn formed not just the basis of the diet, but the entire diet in some localities. The reason is that the Aztecs ate many other foods which provided the elements lacking in corn.

Corn was made into a porridge called *atole* which was seasoned with pimiento or honey or a syrup made from the maguey cactus. *Tamales* are envelopes of steamed cornmeal stuffed with various vegetables and meats. The Aztecs made them with more than 40 different shapes and fillings. They might be stuffed with mushrooms, fruits, fish, rabbit, beans, turkey eggs, green or red peppers. There were also tamales stuffed with frogs, snails, beeswax, tadpoles or axolotls (the immature form of salamander that looks a little like a newt).

The Aztec city of Tenochtitlan was beside a lake. The Indians used every product that could be found on or in the lake, including fish, shrimp and the larvae of water flies. They skimmed the clumps of insect eggs off the surface of the water and ate them like caviar. Axolotls served with yellow peppers were considered a dish for the king's table. There were also plenty of waterfowl on the lake and around it were deer, peccary, rabbits, gophers and pigeons. Many kinds of fruit were grown by the farmers, plus tomatoes, amaranth, avocadoes, several kinds of beans, mushrooms, leafy greens and grubs from the leaves of the maguey cactus.

Wild turkeys had been domesticated and were raised on farms. And dogs were fattened for food and considered good eating. The first meal was served about 10 in the morning—probably a dish of corn porridge or mush, as we would call it. The main meal was at noon and was usually followed by a siesta. The noon meal might be tortillas or corn griddlecakes and beans covered with tomato sauce and chili peppers. Supper was eaten just before bedtime. It might consist of another bowl of gruel made from sage or corn or amaranth. Rolled *tortillas* were used as spoons.

As one might expect, rich people had much more variety in their meals. They could afford pineapples, chocolate, oysters, crabs, turtles and sea fish brought from the coast. Here are some of the delicacies which might have graced the table of Montezuma, the Aztec emperor of Mexico who was captured by the Spaniard Cortez in the early 16th century.

According to reports of a contemporary observer, he "sat behind a screen at a table covered with fine white cloths. Four clean and beautiful girls brought water for his hands while others brought maize (corn) cakes. . . . For each meal his cooks made him more than 30 different dishes prepared according to their style and customs, and underneath them they put small earthenware braziers to prevent the food from getting cold. They cooked more than 300 plates of the food the Great Montezuma was going to eat and over 1,000 more for the guard."

Some of the dishes were: locusts prepared with sage, fish with chili peppers and tomatoes, prickly pears (*opuntia*) with fish eggs, frogs with green chilies, venison with red chilies, tomatoes and ground squash seeds. Also served were duck stewed in a pot, and gourd seeds, roasted and salted as we prepare our peanuts. Montezuma then had some fruit for dessert, along with some chocolate. After watching some entertainment and having a smoke, he retired.

Chocolate was prepared by pounding cacao nuts, then boiling them in water with a little corn flour. The oil was skimmed off, strained into a vessel and whipped into a froth which gradually dissolved in the mouth. Chocolate was generally drunk cold, and often flavored with honey, vanilla or spices. Delicious? The Aztecs made a dish of venison served in a chocolate sauce with red peppers and herbs. The chocolate gave the dish a flavor much like wine.

Corn was planted by the Aztecs from March until early May, in time to catch the rains that started in May and ended in July or August. The best corn was put away for the next year's seed, after being taken to the temple of the corn goddess Chicomecoatl for blessing.

A present-day Mayan family of five eats about six and a half pounds of corn every day, says Warwick Bray. An Aztec family might have had three acres of land on which they could have raised 2,500 pounds of corn a year, along with the other foods they needed. Today in Mayan territory a family may have 10 to 12 acres and produce twice as much corn as the family needs. Squash and beans were, and are, planted in the fields with the corn, the squash to shield the tender young corn shoots, the beans to climb the stalks as they grow higher. The beans help to contribute nitrogen to the soil and protein to the Aztec and modern Mayan meals.

Other important crops were *chia* (*Salvia Hispanica*) and amaranth. The *chia* seeds were made into gruel or porridge. The Aztecs also got oil from the seeds. Amaranth (*Amaranthus Paniculatus*) produced tiny seeds which were parched and ground, then used for gruel or dough. The importance of amaranth as a crop depended on its date of maturation. It ripened at the end of the rainy season and before corn could be harvested. So in case the corn crop failed, there were plenty of amaranth seeds on hand to tide the community over until other foods were available. Amaranth seeds were such an important crop that we are told over 150,000 bushels of them were sent as tribute every year to Montezuma.

The maguey cactus (*Agave Atrovirens*) grows wild on dry infertile soil. According to Bray it endures extremes of weather and rainfall and requires 10 years to mature. All of the maguey was used by the Aztecs. A juice which oozed out when the flower heads were cut was stored in skins or gourds, used as a sweetener or as a medicine and also fermented into *octli,* a beverage which, now called *pulque,* is still popular in Mexico. A single maguey cactus gives up to 15 pints of sap a day.

Bees were domesticated. A farmer going out to take the honey might have addressed his bees thus, to explain his action, "I, who come to do this unfriendly act, come compelled by necessity, since I am poor and miserable; thus I come only to seek my maintenance, and so let none of you be afraid nor be frightened of me. I am only going to take you so that you can see my sister the goddess of Xochiquetzel, she who is called the Precious Branch." Early Mexicans

59

also ate the larvae of the bees.

The Aztecs hunted and fished for white-tailed deer, peccary, rabbits, coyotes, armadillos, gophers, iguana lizards, wild guinea pigs and little birds, quail, pigeons, waterfowl. They set traps and weirs for fresh and salt-water fish. They ate many insects. Grasshoppers were thrown into large vats of boiling grease where the horny parts floated to the surface of the oil and the delicious edible meat stayed behind to be "French fried."

Beans were used by all the early civilizations of Mexico, Central and South America. They had lima and scarlet-runner beans, white, black, pea beans, black-eyed beans, kidney beans, tiny beans, jet black or purple, big flat beans with edible pods and beans with slender edible pods enclosing seeds hardly larger than BB shot.

And the Indians of North and South America counted as "beans" many other foods which we do not eat today. The seeds of the beautiful wild lupines were "beans" to them. Many trees of the locust family bear edible "beans." In Chile the seeds of the algarroba tree (*Ceratonia siliqua*) are eaten as beans. This is the carob tree, one of the few exotic plants with which we are familiar, since carob flour is becoming a popular health store item as a substitute for commercially-processed chocolate. The yam-bean or sincama (*Cacara tuberosa*) of tropical America has edible pods containing "beans," as well as a large turnip-like root which is also edible.

Peanuts are often found on ancient Peruvian pottery. Graves in Incan and pre-Incan time were furnished with a ration of peanuts to nourish the dead person on the journey to heaven. Many times peanuts which have lain in such graves are in an excellent state of preservation, after thousands of years, since the containers were carefully sealed to keep out air and moisture. The Indians had many varieties of peanuts and probably ate them almost the way we do. They also made peanut butter. The Incan name for peanuts is *mani,* which means ground-seed. Peanuts, of course, grow in the soil on the tips of branches of the plants, which bury themselves in the ground.

Vanilla is the seed pod of a climbing orchid (*Vanilla planifolia*) which grows mostly in Southeastern Mexico. Like *manioc,* the vanilla seed pod is inedible and flavorless until it is processed. We do not know how the early Indians discovered ways to change this plain brown seed pod into the fragrant food which today flavors delicacies all over the world.

The pods are picked with great care, for they are easily damaged. Verrill tells us most of the labor is done by Indians whose ancestors raised and cured vanilla for Montezuma and his family. The pods are spread on blankets and exposed to the sun, then rolled up in the blanket at night and in wet weather. The pods darken and wrinkle. In a week or two they are cured—an even, brown or nearly black leathery pod, tough and pliable, with a strong vanilla fragrance. Then they must be dried, very slowly, for six to ten weeks. Don't mistake synthetic vanilla for the real thing. The synthetic stuff is made of woodpulp paste.

Reay Tannahill in *Food and History,* tells the almost unbelievable story of *zamia* bread which, she says, was a specialty of the Taino tribes who met Columbus. The bread was made by grating the stems of the zamia plant, then shaping the pulp into balls which were left in the sun for two or three days until they began to rot, turn black and become infested with worms. Then they were flattened into cakes and baked on a griddle. The Taino alleged that if they were eaten before they were black and full of worms, they would kill the eater. And this is so. The pulp must be thoroughly fermented or washed, or it is toxic.

61

In case you have a yen to try this delectable morsel, *zamia* trees grow in Florida, the West Indies, Mexico and Guatemala.

We do not know the origin of pineapples but they were grown by pre-Incan people in the lowlands of Central and South America. The finest of these fruits were grown in the West Indies. Nobody who buys pineapples in a modern American city has any idea of what the luscious fruits taste like when they are picked ripe, for they must be picked green to be shipped to our stores. Among the Indians, and among early settlers in our country, the pineapple was the symbol of hospitality. This explains the carved pineapples found on Colonial furniture, bed posts and newel posts.

In the same botanical family as potatoes are two other vegetables which originated in South America—tomatoes and peppers. All of them are members of the deadly nightshade family, but they are not poisonous. Wild tomatoes may have appeared first as weeds in the Indians' corn fields. Pre-Incan Indians grew them and probably developed them from small insignificant berries into fleshy fruits by the time European conquerors arrived in the New World. They were taken to Europe and looked upon with suspicion, for it was widely believed that they were poisonous. Italians were the first Europeans to adopt them with consequences everyone knows who has ever tasted spaghetti or lasagna. What would the Italian cuisine be without tomatoes?

Peppers (the *Capsicum* family) were called *aji* (pronounced "ah-hee") by the Incans. South Americans have many varieties from very sweet green ones to extremely hot chili peppers and cayenne, which is hottest of the hot. Verrill says he saw peppers of many shapes, colors, flavors and sizes in his travels in South and Central America: round, conical, flat, twisted, carrot-like, pear-shaped, dark red, scarlet, yellow or almost white. They vary in size from very large ones to the tiny pea-like varieties. The little ones are the hottest. Verrill is certain that no Northerner could ever endure the agonies of eating one of the hot varieties, but in many parts of the tropics the Indians are very fond of them. Mayan children munch on the fiery little peppers as we might eat peanuts or popcorn and apparently enjoy them.

Why this delight in something so peppery? We don't know. Possibly they stimulate the digestive organs and the liver and may thus improve general health. Perhaps by heating up the insides, they make people in tropical countries feel cooler. Perhaps they help to conceal the taste of spoiled or rancid food.

High in the Sierra Madre Mountains in Mexico lives a small nation, the Tarahumara Indians. So remarkable are the hearts of these people that they can run 100 miles or more without stopping and with no discomfort. Equally amazing is their psychological and cultural adjustment, says an article in the *Journal of the American Medical Association* for June 2, 1969. Two University of Oklahoma researchers studied the Indians to discover the effects of such incredible exertion on their hearts and circulatory systems. They reported on their findings at a symposium. They studied eight male runners from 18 to 48 years old. Their diastolic blood pressure had decreased midpoint of a 28-mile kick-ball race. Pulse rates had risen from 120 to 155. They lost an average of five pounds each during the race.

"These marathon demonstrations of really phenomenal endurance are convincing evidence that most of us, brought up in our comfortable and sedentary civilizations, actually develop and use only a fraction of our potential cardiac reserve," said Dr. Dale Groom. X-rays of the Indians' chests showed hearts of normal size, not the enlarged "athlete's hearts" with which we are familiar.

In all the Indians, skeletal muscles give out before the

heart muscle does. None of the Indians could remember any occasion on which a runner dropped out of a race because of shortness of breath or chest pain. They, however, get leg cramps and they have urinary problems which may arise from the kidneys shutting down because of the exertion.

The Tarahumara Indians live on what American home economists would probably describe as a "poor diet." They have corn, squash, beans, and "wild plants," with occasional game and fish. They plant gardens and raise crops, but they are also semi-nomadic. So probably they eat much the same kind of diet we have described for most South American Indians. The corn and beans eaten together make up complete vegetable protein. The squash contributes vitamin A, the wild plants vitamin C and A. This is, in essence, a high protein diet, albeit a sparse one. There is little carbohydrate and certainly no refined carbohydrate or concentrated sugars of any kind. According to the *JAMA* article, conditions are very primitive and 80 percent of the children die before the age of six because of malnutrition, infections and parasites.

The great distances between individual families "undoubtedly cause people to be keenly aware of their need for each other and appreciative of the value of persons," a university professor of Psychiatry and Behavioral Sciences told the symposium. They have a quiet dignity, respect for one another, good humor and helpfulness toward strangers. Most remarkable, says the *Journal,* is that interpersonal or intergroup violence is virtually unknown in spite of a highly structured family life and fierce local loyalties. They are great competitors, but trading is fair and honest. Almost nobody steals. There are ceremonial drinking parties, but alcoholism is unknown, as is divorce.

Faced with such beautiful people, embodying most of the qualities modern industrial societies pretend to venerate but actually outrage, physicians are in a quandary as to just what is their duty toward these people. If modern medicine brings them antibiotics, prenatal care, vitamins, vaccinations and drugs to prevent parasites, babies will stop dying and the number of Indians will increase to such an extent that their mountain home will not be able to support them. It is unlikely that they will agree to contraceptives.

The physicians, who are even now sending in drugs and vaccines, are asking themselves, "In two generations of ten-child families, the ancient and beautiful culture of the Tarahumara could be destroyed. Should we rush in to save the Tarahumara babies or should we continue to let them die?" Modern physicians and philosophers have not as yet come to any workable answer to this question.

And from Peru, we have reports of another Indian nation, living in much the same general environment, but with completely different personalities. One anthropologist believes he knows why. Dr. Ralph Bolton, of Pomona College, California, recently returned from Peru where he spent five years living with the Qolla Indians in a remote mountainous area. He believes he has found a connection between the hostile, aggressive behavior of these Peruvians and low blood sugar levels. This is a condition which can masquerade as many different physical diseases.

Frequently it involves heavy sweating, fainting spells, headaches, hunger, irritability or nervousness. Many of the unpleasant feelings that plague dieters on reducing diets low in protein may be associated with the low blood sugar condition such diets produce. And the low blood sugar may be one reason why such diets are so hard to maintain.

The Qolla have no problems with reducing diets. Instead, like poor people in our own country, they suffer gross dietary deficiencies from eating a low-protein, high-carbohydrate diet, consisting mostly of potatoes, barley, oats and *quinoa,* a grain which will grow at high altitudes. In addition, they live in a hostile environment. The terrain is mountainous and barren. The climate is erratic, with hail, drought and frost, which means that harvests are likely to be uncertain and scanty.

Dr. Bolton describes the Qolla as people who enjoy a good fight, "because it makes one feel better." Very hostile and aggressive, these two million people are pretty regularly "spoiling for a fight" just for the heck of it. The anthropologist believes that the combination of circumstances— inadequate diet, overpopulation, scarcity of land, unpredictable weather and lack of enough oxygen (because of the altitude at which they live) may be the starting points for the development of low blood sugar levels.

He found the Qolla to be "strutting, swaggering individuals," especially when they are drunk. They will go to outrageous lengths to insult others and precipitate a fight, sometimes indulging in monologues describing their own ferocity while laughing at the puniness of their enemies. Threats produce such sensitivity in the Qolla that just the phrase "you'll see" can be construed as a verbal attack. Saying "I am a man" immediately implies that others are not men, so whoever is within hearing distance takes this sentence as an insult and a battle ensues.

Fighting and killing are not the only forms of aggression. Injuries, insults, stealing, rape, arson, abortion, slander, failure to pay debts, land ownership disputes and homicide are common. In one village of 1,200 Qolla, Dr. Bolton found that half of the heads of households had been involved, directly or indirectly, in homicide cases. The rate of homicide among the Qolla is 50 per 100,000—far higher than in almost any other group in the world.

Surprisingly enough, the traditional philosophy of the Qolla is far from aggressive. They believe in the Christian virtues of charity, compassion and cooperation with others.

And they almost never perceive any discrepancy between their beliefs and their actions. Other anthropologists have always found the Qolla to be "the meanest and most unlikeable people on earth." Traditionally this has been excused on the basis of the extreme hardness of their lives and the fact that they have usually lived under domination by one or another conquering nation.

Dr. Bolton believes this is not the complete story. Other nations living under harsh conditions do not have the same characteristics of aggression and hostility. True, the Qolla have been conquered many times, but, he says, they tend to ignore outside influences, even conquerors, and continue to go about their own hostile pursuits. They live in a constant state of anarchy.

The anthropologist had read about hypoglycemia, or low blood sugar, and decided to test some of the Qolla. He did blood sugar analyses of all adult males in one village and found that blood sugar levels were low in 50 percent of them. Interestingly enough, they chew the coca leaf. Coca leaves are the substance from which cocaine is made. Their action is similar to that of opium, although somewhat less narcotic. They deaden the sense of taste and anesthetize the membranes of the stomach, thus cutting off hunger.

So it is possible, under the influence of coca, to go without food or consciousness of needing it for as long as three days. But the body starves, as might be expected. Continual heavy use of coca produces body wasting, mental failure, insomnia, circulatory weakness and dyspepsia. However, under the influence of the drug, addicts are able to perform great feats of endurance.

In addition to chewing coca leaves, the Qolla use a lot of alcohol, again, Dr. Bolton believes, in an effort to bring blood sugar levels up to a comfortable condition. Alcohol does this in susceptible persons, then causes these levels to drop far below normal, bringing on the same symptoms the alcoholic has tried to overcome. So it becomes necessary to have another and yet another drug of some kind, merely to keep going with any comfort.

Very little research has been done on low blood sugar in relation to aggression. During the 1940's a number of American doctors proposed the theory that low blood sugar is the leading cause of many acts of criminal violence, even murder.

Hypoglycemia may be a factor, says Dr. Bolton, in some cases of criminal behavior in "civilized" societies. An otherwise normal-appearing person may be driven to commit atrocities by his body's urge to restore a proper blood sugar balance. Aware that the body will go to extraordinary lengths to repair a malfunction within itself, Dr. Bolton believes that the Qolla are forced into aggressive behavior by their physical condition.

Low blood sugar conditions are intolerable to the human body. Death can result from extremes of this condition, as diabetics well know. Dr. Bolton believes that through aggressive thought and activity, the Qolla unconsciously try to raise their blood sugar levels to a comfortable point. Psychologically, they force themselves into a state of anger so their internal organs can temporarily restore a proper bodily balance.

He believes that hypoglycemia or low blood sugar should be suspected when studying social conflict and behavior patterns of any "peasant" culture. We wonder why he specifies "peasant," since many of the circumstances he outlines appear to be just as prevalent on city streets, where badly nourished people commit crimes to get money for drugs, where people go berserk, within hours of apparent sanity, and kill wildly and indiscriminately anyone they can reach with a gun.

He goes on to say, "The question of peasant personality should be looked at again, since many of the same factors which serve as stressors for the Qolla are present in most peasant societies. Research on this topic might be carried out in American ghettos and other poverty areas where high levels of stress are found."

Dr. Bolton does not mention it, but obviously one form of stress on city streets must be the low blood sugar caused by a deficient diet, overbalanced with sweets and carbohydrates—especially the concentrated sugar in soft drinks and candy which make up such a large part of the diet of so many people.

Dr. Bolton wants to go on studying this line of thought. He says his study opens up many research possibilities, for example, detailed studies of the relationship between coca chewing and other drug use and hypoglycemia, the relationship between alcohol consumption and hypoglycemia, and the consequences of hypoglycemia for other psychological processes such as perception, memory and cognition. He believes, too, that a comparative study of aggressive and peaceful societies may eventually lead to a significant anthropological contribution to a general theory of human conflict and aggression. A full account of Dr. Bolton's work was published in *Ethnology,* Volume XII, 1973.

In primitive Eskimo societies, conditions of environmental stress are also extreme. The cold, the darkness, the continual battle for food must indeed be among the most difficult ways of life anywhere in the world. Primitive Eskimos eat a diet consisting almost entirely of protein and fat.

Yet primitive Eskimos are so far removed from violence that there is no word for "war" in any Eskimo language. Explorers have tried to make their Eskimo friends understand what is meant by war. The Eskimos simply refuse to believe that any human being could possibly go out and kill total strangers for any reason whatsoever. We know of no blood sugar studies among primitive Eskimos. But it appears that their blood sugar levels must be very well regulated. Their kind of diet practically guarantees this.

And then there are the residents of Vilcabamba in Ecuador. One hundred years of healthy life are considered not very long by these people who have achieved, among gerontologists, about the same stature in health and longevity as the Hunzas and the remarkable people who live high in the Caucasus Mountains of the U.S.S.R.

Specialists in old age are studying these people with great interest to determine if they can pinpoint just why and how they live such remarkably healthy long lives. Do they inherit some magical combination of glands and enzymes? Is it their surroundings, their diet, the amount of exercise they get?

In *New Scientist* for February 2, 1973, Dr. David Davies, a member of the Unit of Gerontology at University College, London, describes his encounter with these inhabitants of a South American Shangri-la. He talked to some 24 old folks, their birthdates well authenticated by church records, all of them alert, bright, active, with excellent teeth. He gives us a photograph of José David who, at the age of 142, was busily hoeing his corn.

Meals in Vilcabamba are "frugal." They consist of soup made of grain, corn, *yuca* (*manioc*), beans and potatoes. The people eat a considerable amount of vegetables, says Dr. Davies, along with no more than an ounce of meat a week. They also have oranges and bananas, and "a little" refined sugar. The diet contains little fat.

The available milk is almost always made into cheese. A reservoir has been built to supply them with drinking water, but they prefer to drink water from the nearby river, as they always have. Scientists from an Ecuador university are investigating the minerals in the water to see if they might influence this great record of longevity.

And now for the most astonishing news of all—the old folks of Vilcabamba drink two to four cups of homemade rum every day and smoke from 40 to 60 cigarettes. The rum is unrefined, made from raw sugar, the cigarettes are made from their own home grown tobacco and rolled in corn husks.

Dr. Davies believes it is quite possible these old folks live to such a great age simply because they are wanted and feel useful. They have jobs to do, gardens to care for, and a definite contribution to make to the welfare of the community. He says that this perhaps gives them a feeling of usefulness because they are contributing to the whole family—"a factor which sociologists are increasingly realizing to be of importance to mental, if not physical, well being."

Alexander Leaf, M.D., the Massachusetts gerontologist, travelled to Vilcabamba and reported his observations in *Nutrition Today* for September/October, 1973. He compared the environment of the very old people he studied there, with that of Hunza and the Georgian Republic.

Vilcabamba is high in the mountains and the people work very, very hard at subsistence farming. Tobacco and sugarcane are the principal crops. Although the villagers smoke, there is no certain information on how many of them inhale. They engage in "vigorous physical exercise."

Dr. Leaf's description of hygiene in this remote spot boggles the mind. The residents do all their laundry and bathing in the river from which they get their drinking water. (Of course they may not drink much water, since they drink so much rum.) He inquired about the bathing habits of the villagers. Some had not bathed for several years. One had been unwashed for ten years.

Most of them live in mud huts with dirt floors and

chickens and pigs in the house with them. Infant mortality is high. But the number of old people is astonishingly great. Nine of the population of 810 are 100 years old. Miguel Carpio, the oldest when Dr. Leaf was there, is 121. José Toledo is 109. They are both mentally alert and well preserved physically. All the old folks were born locally. Dr. Leaf believes that genetic factors must somehow play an important role in this phenomenon.

The Vilcabamba diet averages only 1,200 calories daily with a maximum of 1,360. The daily protein intake is 35 to 38 grams. The recommended allowance in the U.S.A. is 56 grams for adults. The fat intake is only 12 to 19 grams and there are 200 to 260 grams of carbohydrate or starch. About 12 grams of protein daily come from animal sources, all the rest is vegetable. Obesity is unknown.

The *New York Dental Journal,* December, 1965, carried an article by H. H. Neumann and N. DiSalvo of Columbia University, in which these two dental experts sought to explain the absence of decayed teeth among primitive people and the rapid onset of decay once a "modern" diet is adopted. The low rate of decay among primitive people cannot be ascribed to racial immunity, heredity, oral hygiene, climatic conditions, or fluoride in the drinking water, they tell us.

What then? Well, it seems that many primitive people chew hard things—"high-chewing loads," as the experts put it. In Mexico the toasted *haba* beans (lima beans) are eaten. Among other people unground betel nuts are chewed, bones are cracked with the teeth, as well as the shells of nuts and the shells of crustaceans. A hard, crusted bread is eaten in Southern Italy and Eastern Europe.

These Columbia researchers say that "compression stress" may alter the molecular structure of the enamel, thus making it more resistant to noxious agents in the mouth.

Well and good. There seems to be no doubt that chewing crusty, crunchy, chewy foods is good for the health of teeth and gums alike. It exercises gums and apparently keeps teeth well fixed in their proper places. But unfortunately, these researchers do not point out, in their theorizing, that really primitive people have no access to the foods which have been shown, in hundreds of careful laboratory experiments, to create rampant tooth decay among animals as well as people—the refined and processed carbohydrates which stick around the teeth. Especially sugar.

The Traditional Diet of Eskimos Is Meat and Fish and That's about All

Anyone who doubts the benefits of a wholly natural, unprocessed, unrefined, unchemicalized diet and the immeasurable damage that can be done by the typical modern diet eaten by Western industrialized nations, should study the facts carefully laid out and beautifully illustrated in *Nutrition Today,* November/December, 1971.

"Few if any population groups have ever experienced such rapid changes as the Eskimos, in their way of living and their diets. The effects of their changed food habits on growth and health are evident on all sides," says Dr. Otto Schaefer, M.D.

His article goes on to say that when Eskimos give up their nomadic lives and settle down in towns sponsored and employed by white men, remarkable changes soon take place. Eskimo children grow faster and taller and reach puberty at an earlier age. Their teeth decay. Eskimo women develop gall bladder problems and some member of the family will almost certainly develop another of the chronic degenerative diseases well known among white populations. Dr. Schaefer, a long-time student of the Canadian Arctic, is deeply concerned for the welfare of the Eskimos.

He reports that the diseases of civilization follow directly upon the exposure of the Eskimos to white culture—both the changes in eating habits and changes in the diet eaten by the Eskimo when he moves to a settlement. In earlier times, the diet of these inland Eskimos consisted almost entirely of game and fish. The daily food intake was almost entirely animal protein: mammals both large and small, many kinds of fish and birds, along with some seasonal berries, roots, leafy greens and seaweed.

In a diet such as this, carbohydrate is almost completely lacking. The very small amount available was considered a great delicacy by the Eskimos. It was the natural sugar, glycogen, found in the livers of the animals they ate, and a bit of carbohydrate found beneath the skin of the whale. Neither carbohydrate was easily assimilated.

In the mid-1950's a string of military and civilian airports was built across the Canadian Arctic. Attracted by new jobs, new houses and schools, the Eskimos abandoned their nomadic lives and went to live in the settlements.

In earlier days, Eskimos ate most of their meat raw. This required much vigorous chewing. Women also had the job of chewing on tough animal skins to render them pliant for boots and clothing. In the settlements, the men now eat at the company cafeteria. They are getting fat. Their teeth are rotting. The women, who no longer have need to fish, tan skins or sew clothing, spend their time at the movies, eat a lot of candy, drink a lot of coke and suffer from many hitherto unknown disorders, the most noticeable being rampant tooth decay.

In earlier times the Eskimo ate perhaps 318 grams of protein a day, while his present diet gives him about 100 grams. From a diet in which carbohydrate was very scarce, he has gone, in one generation, to a diet *which includes almost 200 pounds of white sugar a year*—an appalling amount of readily absorbed sugar.

Dr. Schaefer points out that, while urban populations in Western countries have also increased enormously their consumption of sugar, this has happened over a century. But with the Eskimos it has happened within the short period of 20 years or so.

Aside from tooth decay, what are some of the diseases commonplace among Western nations which are now becoming widespread plagues among the Eskimos? They are diabetes, hardening of the arteries, heart attacks, obesity, gallstones and acne.

"We have reason to believe," says Dr. Schaefer, "that the great and rapid increase in consumption of sucrose (sugar)—especially if taken, as is increasingly the case, without preceding meat meals—may have serious metabolic-endocrine repercussions."

The "repercussions" he refers to are effects which disrupt blood sugar levels, glands and the entire digestive and assimilative process by which the body handles food. The high sugar content stimulates glands, over-producing insulin and causing rapid growth. If the Eskimos were still living lives of extreme physical exertion, as they used to, this physical activity might "cushion" the effects of the shock to glands. But Eskimos are becoming more and more sedentary, just as the rest of us are.

Dr. Schaefer says that the metabolic-endocrine consequences of wild blood sugar fluctuations are present. He believes, he says, that they are related to many other disorders which are presently afflicting people in the industrialized parts of the world.

Eskimo children now grow faster and taller. The girls reach puberty at an earlier age—a situation "directly related to the increased consumption of sugar without increased protein," says Dr. Schaefer. Diabetes is not yet widely prevalent among the Eskimos, but in some parts of the community the disease is already three times more prevalent than it was ten years ago. A five times greater incidence of circulatory disorders is showing up in Eskimos who have lived the "civilized" life for more than 10 years. Rotten teeth and the tendency to circulatory troubles appear to correlate.

There is a significant increase in the cholesterol and other fatty content of blood among Eskimos on the high-carbohydrate diet and a great increase in the number who are obese. But obesity and overweight are confined mostly to those under 40 years of age, those who have eaten lots of carbohydrate almost all their lives. The incidence of gall bladder troubles and acne is steadily rising. Dr. Schaefer laments the fact that the Eskimos themselves blame the pimply skin of their children on the soda, candy and chocolate they eat *as if they were addicted.*

In many a modern medical journal you will find assurances that diet has nothing at all to do with the present-day epidemic of acne in the U.S.A. Dr. Schaefer wonders what old time Northerners would say to this, for they know well that acne and other skin disorders were unknown to Eskimos eating their traditional diets.

Finally, a basic difference in the way babies are fed has resulted in higher infant mortality and a fifty percent jump in the birthrate. Eskimo mothers traditionally nursed their children for as long as three years. In addition to mother's milk, the baby got supplements of raw meat and fish. The next child was not born until this lengthy lactation period was over. So a self-regulating birth control was practiced which kept Eskimo families small. It also kept Eskimo babies healthy.

As nursing bottles and prepared formulas became available in the settlements, Eskimo mothers began to feed their babies with these artificial formulas. The birth rate began to rise, for the three-year sterile period no longer prevailed. And the infants' immunity to many diseases granted by mother's milk disappeared as well.

Dr. Schaefer tells us that a careful survey of infant mortality and disease turned up the fact that bottle-fed children have a higher incidence of diseases of the digestive tract and also respiratory and middle-ear diseases, and anemia. Earache—an infected inner ear—has become one of the most widespread disorders of bottle-fed Eskimo children.

The changed feeding practices and what Dr. Schaefer calls "the extraordinary perversion of the female breast from a nutritional organ to a sex symbol, which is so typical of Western civilization" have brought about vast changes in health, not only during infancy but far beyond. Allergies and auto-immune diseases are far more prevalent in adults who were bottle-fed as babies.

Mothers suffer, too, Dr. Schaefer says, because of the frustration of the natural function of a human organ—the breast. In Eskimos, as well as other people, the incidence of breast cancer appears to tie in directly with the period of lactation. The longer babies are nursed, the less breast cancer appears. Among Eskimo mothers nursing their babies in the traditional way, breast cancer was unknown.

Dr. Schaefer speaks of the "frightening speed" with which all these disasters have overtaken the Eskimos, as a result of abandoning their old ways and taking up our customs—chiefly the food which has been denatured to such an extent that the body simply cannot handle it healthfully.

Dr. Schaefer believes that the Eskimos' experience is sound evidence that many of the diseases of civilization which puzzle our best medical specialists have a nutritional basis. Pointing out the importance of physical exercise, he said, in a letter to *The Lancet*, April 14, 1973, that semi-nomadic Eskimos have lower cholesterol levels than those

Eskimos in younger age-groups who live in towns.

Vigorous exercise does indeed lower cholesterol levels. The low pulse rates and blood pressures of long-distance runners and mountain climbers suggest the direct influence of exercise on blood fats and blood pressure.

The Eskimos of Alaska who were studied by Dr. Weston Price and reported on in *Nutrition and Physical Degeneration* had a native diet which consisted almost entirely of meat from sea mammals and fish. They dried their fish in large quantities for winter use. Fish were also eaten frozen. Seal meat and seal oil were used in abundance whenever seal could be found. Caribou (reindeer) meat was another delicacy. In every case, the organs of the animals were considered especially valuable.

Of vegetable foods these Eskimos had only a few berries which were eaten in summer or stored in fat for winter use. They also robbed the nests of tundra mice for a ground nut. They ate certain water grasses, plants and bulbs. But the bulk of the diet was meat, fish and fish eggs.

Obviously the diet of primitive Eskimos contained relatively enormous amounts of fat which they loved and ate regularly. Yet, until they began to eat "store-bought" food they never suffered from the circulatory (heart and artery) plagues which are epidemics in all modern Western countries. So how can "too much fat" be incriminated as the only, or even the main, cause of these modern plagues? If fat is indeed the villain of the piece, why didn't fatty food affect the Eskimos the same way it is supposed to affect the Wall Street businessman? Nutrition experts who are wedded to the theory of dietary fat as the main cause of circulatory disorders are strangely silent on the subject of Eskimo diets.

Dr. Price visited Ketchikan, Alaska, where the variety of sea foods, especially salmon, seemed almost limitless. But he found many Indians eating the cheap store food. In one

80

settlement he found that 46.6 percent of all teeth he examined were riddled with tooth decay. Many people were ill with tuberculosis and arthritis. At Juneau 75 percent of the people in the hospital had tuberculosis and fifty percent of all patients were under 21 years old! Almost 40 percent of all teeth were decayed. At Sitka a similar situation prevailed.

In Anchorage, he studied one family in which the mother and son were living entirely on moose and deer meat, fresh and dried fish plus some cranberries and a few vegetables. The 63 year-old mother was entirely free from tooth decay. Her son had one cavity. The daughter of the family had married a white man. They had chosen to live on processed food, including large amounts of white bread, syrup and potatoes. Twenty-two of her teeth were destroyed by decay. Tooth decay was rampant in her children whose jaws and face structure were also deformed.

Comparing the native diet of Eskimos and the diet which Western man brought to this ancient culture, Dr. Price found that the food of the native Eskimos contained 5.4 times more calcium than the "store-bought" food, 1.5 times more iron, 7.9 times more magnesium, 1.8 times more copper, 49 times more iodine, and at least 10 times more of the fat soluble vitamins, such as A and D.

A modern London physician reporting on his sojourn among Eskimos at North West River, said that he found few cancers, little arthritis or cardiac disease. But, since civilization had brought "the blessings" of soft drinks and candy, the children were already beginning to show overweight and tooth destruction.

One of the all-time great experts on the Far North was Dr. Vilhjalmur Stefansson, who spent much of his life there. He was also very knowledgeable in the field of nutrition. He came back from the North one day to challenge the A.M.A. and every orthodox authority on diet by claiming in a published article that human beings could live healthfully on nothing but fatty meat.

He proved it, too, in a closely supervised test lasting for more than a year, during which time he lived at Bellevue Hospital in New York and ate nothing but fatty mutton— as much as he wanted. He was given every imaginable test at the end of this time and was found to be in as good, or better, shape than when he began the test.

He has this to say about Eskimo food in his book *The Friendly Arctic,* "Questions are frequently put to me as to whether caribou meat or musk-ox meat or bear meat or seal meat is good eating, and then I struggle against impatience, for underlying the query is a fundamental misunderstanding of human tastes and prejudices in food. A rule with no more exceptions than ordinary rules is that people like the sort of food to which they are accustomed. An American will tell you that he can eat white bread every day but that he gets tired of rice if he eats it more than once or twice a month, while a Chinaman may think that rice is an excellent food for every day but that white bread soon palls. An Englishman will tell you that beef is the best meat in the world, while in Iceland or in Tibet you will learn that beef is all right now and then, but mutton is the only meat of which you will never tire. . . . The Eskimos of Prince Albert Sound who on their winter hunts in Banks Island live for several months each year nearly exclusively on polar bear meat, are very fond of it . . ."

He describes the choicest parts of caribou meat. It is interesting that some cuts which we prize most highly are fed to the dogs by the Eskimos. The head is best, they think, and, except for marrow, the most delicious fat is behind the eyes. Then they find the tongue most appealing, then brisket, ribs and vertebrae. In serving all these parts, the outer meat is removed and given to the dogs, while the Eskimos eat only the meat nearest the bones. Then hearts, kidneys and neck meat are eaten. The hams, some of the entrails and the tenderloin are considered food for dogs.

Dr. Stefansson's ideas on fat-eating are considered revolutionary today, at a time when the word "cholesterol" brings nightmares to millions of people trying to avoid circulatory troubles. He says that the preferences of various groups of people for different kinds of fat are especially interesting, for in our times Europeans and Americans have allowed sugar to occupy the chief place where gourmet tastes are concerned. He believes that no one who has been brought up on a typical modern diet, a large part of which consists of sugar and starch, can possibly delight in the fine shades of difference between different kinds of fat. But this power comes very soon irrespective of climate to anyone who lives on unseasoned animal foods exclusively, he tells us.

C. Van Valin in *Eskimoland Speaks,* recounts his experience eating *muktuk,* the black skin of the whale which, he says, looks like a rubber boot heel. It has the flavor of beechnuts and is excellent eating, either cooked or raw. The Eskimos eat it before any other part of whale meat, along with a half inch of blubber with each bite, for lubrication. Blubber on a medium-sized whale is about 18 inches thick and is not solid fat, but fibrous. It is a beautiful rosy pink color, sweet and juicy, and can be chewed for a long time like chewing gum.

Van Valin says the Eskimos he knew ate fat as the staff of life, as bread is eaten farther south. Each bit of cartilage, each particle of tissue is removed and eaten, bones are then cracked for their marrow. Those without marrow are boiled to remove all fat, which is then eaten. Blood is used for soup. Intestines are cleaned and eaten, either cooked or raw. Salmon is slit from head to tail and hung over poles to dry for winter storage. It is eaten with seal oil.

Says Edward Weyer in his fine book *The Eskimos,* "The salient fact regarding the food of the Eskimos is that they eat practically nothing but meat and fish." Seal meat is most important, then polar bear, then walrus, caribou and whale. Musk ox were eaten before they became scarce. No primitive Eskimo eats much vegetable food—not even that which is available at some seasons. Coronation Gulf Eskimos lived in an area where salmon berries or cloud berries were abundant. Yet it had apparently never occurred to them to eat the berries.

In Alaska Eskimos gather and eat lots of blueberries, heath berries, salmon berries and cranberries, plus a kind of wild sorrel. Young willow leaves are boiled and eaten as well as a plant known as "Eskimo rhubarb," and a small tuberous root called Eskimo potato. Labrador Eskimos eat caribou moss. Other groups eat kelp—both the rubbery stalks and the ribbons. It is considered a medicinal plant, but in times of famine it is regarded as food.

In East Greenland crowberries, stonecrop (sedum) and angelica are eaten. In West Greenland the crowberry or curlewberry is mixed with blubber and eaten. In other northern regions Eskimos eat no vegetable food at all, according to observers. The Polar Eskimos have no such food except for the half-digested contents of caribou stomach which are sometimes frozen and kept for winter use.

Much meat and fish are eaten raw simply because cooking is such a difficult task this far north. There is almost no fuel, so roasting is out of the question. For boiling meat in winter, Eskimos must first melt ice and the only utensil may be a stone pot. So just obtaining enough water takes a long time and much fuel. Blubber lamps are used for cooking in some areas.

Weyer tells us that extravagant statements have been

84

made about the quantity of meat Eskimos eat. He quotes one observer who said that Point Barrow Eskimos ate an average of more than eight pounds of meat daily for almost three months. Another traveller reported 15 pounds per person per day. Others report that only in times of plenty is that much meat available and then only four to eight pounds are eaten.

In *The Life of the Copper Eskimos*, D. Jenness says that there are no set hours for eating. Eskimos eat whenever food is available. Usually these Eskimos have a meal in the morning and another at night, but the time of the second meal depends on when the day's work is finished.

According to Jenness, both men and dogs will starve on a diet of lean meat. Only half the quantity of fat seal meat will keep them well-nourished and satisfied. He says that the Eskimo has no abnormally large appetite. A white man living under the same conditions would eat the same way.

He describes a dinner he ate in an Eskimo hut in 1914: caribou fat, frozen caribou meat, a dried and very mouldy fish and a portion of boiled caribou leg. A strip of blubber about the size of a sugar cube was left on the table inside the hut so that visitors might help themselves to this treat.

Ducks, geese and loons were hunted and eaten in spring and fall. Ptarmigan were found in some regions at almost any time of year. Sea gulls and hawks were occasionally killed and eaten. Children sometimes killed small birds whose skins served as hand towels. Generally speaking, he says, it is in the nature of luxury for an Eskimo to dine off anything but caribou, fish or seal.

Jenness tells us he has seen an Eskimo take a bone from rotten caribou meat cached more than a year before, crack it and eat the marrow with great relish although it was swarming with maggots. They also ate grubs of the warble fly which bore through the skin of caribou in the spring. Their only beverage was water, along with the broth or soup in which meat or fish had been cooked.

Lest we begin to think of Eskimos as blood-thirsty villains bent on destroying all animal life in their area, let us remember that they took only what they had to have to survive. They hunted with a mystical regard for the animals they sought as food. Says Robert G. Williamson in *Archives of Environmental Health* for October, 1968, speaking of the Canadian Northwest Eskimos: "Hunting was a sacred pursuit, central to Eskimo life and interest, and undergirded always with prayers, songs, whispered invocations to the animals hunted, prohibitions and taboos, acts of respect and contrition, ingratiation, gratitude, the wearing of amulets and shamanistic attempts at intercession and manipulation of the elemental powers which so completely governed their lives."

Robert Marshall in *Arctic Village* describes the food eaten in the Kubuk area of Eskimo territory as follows: dried fish, usually cured by stowing it away in the ground, uncleaned. "Fish on top no good," an Eskimo friend told him, "give him to dog. Fish on bottom not so rotten, not so bad him smell him, no need him cook, eat him up."

They ate land game, seal and birds, berries, the roots and leaves of various wild plants, the inner bark of willows, birches and alders, seal oil, seal meat, whales and bear with fish oil to flavor everything, including the berries.

Eskimo ice cream is a great delicacy. Marshall describes how it is made. Fatty marrow from caribou bones is mixed with a great deal of fat and a few blueberries. They are melted together, then removed from the fire and beaten as we would whip cream. Finally the ice cream is allowed to cool and solidify into a white creamy substance speckled with the darker berries. Marshall estimates that the dish of Eskimo ice cream which he sampled consisted of about 70 percent pure fat, ten percent blueberries, ten percent lean meat and ten percent animal hair.

One cannot help but wonder where the Eskimo, on his traditional diet, gets the vitamin C which he needs to protect him from scurvy. For this he must depend on vegetable food and whatever vitamin C is available in the animal livers he eats. In cases of scurvy, according to *Natural History of Arctic America,* they use the stomach of a freshly killed reindeer, with the vegetable contents intact. If the patient is very bad, they bind pieces of the deer's stomach, whale or seal meat around his limbs. If a whale is caught, they thrust the scurvy victim into the carcass of the animal. There seems to be no scientific reason why vitamin C would be made available to any of these procedures except the food in the deer's stomach. But apparently there is enough vitamin C to prevent scurvy in fresh meat which is lightly cooked or eaten raw. Dr. Stefansson never reported any scurvy symptoms during his famous Bellevue Hospital experiment.

Charles Hughes, studying an Eskimo village in the 1950's, gave us exact figures on the amount of "store food" eaten by a number of Eskimos in relation to the amount of traditional food such as reindeer, whale skin (*mangtak*), whale flesh, seal, seal organs, walrus, walrus organs, birds, eggs, fish, greens and seaweeds.

The amounts vary with the seasons and with the time of the arrival of the supply ship bringing in food for the store. Bakers' bread is the one food whose consumption surpasses all others the year round, second only to tea. Other "store foods" are: cereals, dried milk, lard, cheese, canned meat, fruit, macaroni, cocoa, candy, sugar, puddings, jams, jellies and canned vegetables.

He found, he says, a real change in consumption of store food within the past 15 years. He quotes his Eskimo friends as telling him, "We got no food—only store food . . . But when we eat whiteman food, we still hungry." And he tells of some young Eskimo patients in a distant hospital who missed their native food so much that they used to lie awake talking about it before they went to sleep at night. When a whale was killed one May, parents of children away at school or in hospital packaged some of the meat and sent it to them as a great treat, for this was the children's first chance in many years to have a taste of *mangtak*.

William Borders, writing from Resolute, Northwest Territories in *The New York Times,* reported on April 21, 1973, on better but not always happier lives for Canada's native Eskimos and Indians. "The change from within one generation, as abrupt as any on earth, has attracted such a flood of scholars here that in a popular joke one Eskimo asks another, 'Who's your anthropologist?' "

"Our people are being forced off the land they know and love," the head of a Regional Indian Brotherhood told Borders, "and the greedy white man is getting all the gravy. We are finally aware of what the hell's going on and we mean to stop it." Indians and Eskimos, once proud and self-reliant, are now completely dominated by the government and most of them are on welfare.

Borders gives us a glimpse of what alcohol is doing to these erstwhile healthy, self-sufficient people. More than 10 percent of all deaths in one year were caused by accidents or violence related to drinking. "Grotesquely drunken" Eskimos and Indians are familiar sights on any local streets.

What happens to Eskimos when their hunting grounds are forbidden to them is related with passion and fury by Farley Mowat in *The Desperate People.* Mowat has lived for years with the Eskimos and Indians of the Far North. He knows the ecology of that part of the world and how the least intrusion by "civilized" man can destroy the slender thread that holds together all living things on the tundra.

In *The Desperate People,* he describes the Ihalmuit, 49 survivors of a nation which once numbered in the thousands. They have been deported from their own land in what Mowat calls "a long series of errors of neglect, misunderstanding, disinterest and bureaucracy by which one race has inadvertently inflicted physical agony and mental torture upon another."

Traders came looking for the skins of the white fox. They killed caribou for their dogs to eat. They gave the Eskimos guns and the Eskimos killed caribou. No one had ever imagined a time when too many caribou could be killed. But by 1925 these Eskimos were in desperate straits. No caribou migration came through that year and there was almost nothing for them to eat.

"The slaughter of the caribou became a blood-letting," according to Mowat, "on an almost unprecedented scale, not only on the open plains but also in the forests where the majority of the herds wintered . . . Starvation became an annual occurrence . . ." In one area in 1929 an entire band of Eskimos perished and the nearby river is now called The River of Graves.

The few hundred Eskimos left depended on selling white fox pelts to the trappers. But by 1932 there was no market for furs. The trappers left. The Eskimos had their land back again, but it was now a land almost devoid of sustenance. The caribou had not returned. In 1942 one-third of all remaining Eskimos died of starvation.

Mowat says the caribou were doomed by the destruction brought by the white hunter's rifles and unlimited ammunition, as well as the wastage of forests to the south where fires were set by prospectors trying to expose naked rocks, or settlers eager to clear land.

Lichen is the chief food of caribou. When spruce-lichen forests are destroyed by fire, it may take 75 to 100 years for them to be renewed. So the caribou starved and so did the Eskimos who depended upon them. The chain, the link, the balance had been destroyed. The Eskimos were moved by government officials to another location and were told to fish for a living. But they were fully aware that fresh water fish cannot sustain life in the bitter environment of the Far North. "They knew that fish might suffice to keep a man alive if there was nothing else to eat, but only at a fearful cost in the slow wastage of his body," says Mowat.

Mowat went back in 1958 to find his Eskimo friends "unreachable." Their minds were gone, he says. They were crippled and bitter. The remaining Eskimos lived in six tents in a condition bordering on coma.

Such is the saga of "civilized" interference with primitive people. The ancestors of these Eskimos had lived successful'y in this region for thousands of years, surviving well enough in spite of terrible hardships and cold, as well as periods when food was scarce. But they knew how to obtain food and they knew which foods would nourish them. Once this ecology had been destroyed, they perished.

One can only marvel at the casualness with which our Congress permitted the Alaska pipeline to go forward, although they were fully aware of the drastic destruction of this magnificent wilderness area that was certain to follow.

Far Eastern People
Eat Rice and
Many Other Foods

From ancient times the Chinese have had no good opinion of dairy products. Milk, as well as butter, cream and cheese, are simply not part of the Chinese cuisine. They eat little meat as well. Kenneth Scott Latourette in his book *The Chinese, Their History and Culture,* reminds us that not eating much meat is a great advantage in a country where the population is so large that every inch of fertile land counts.

"To use the products of the field directly for human food without the waste of first passing them through the digestive processes of an intermediary animal obviously affects an economy in an area needed to support a given number of human beings," he says. Many modern vegetarians rightly insist on the soundness of their diets on this basis.

Indeed, in her recent book *Diet for a Small Planet,* Frances Moore Lappé analyzes our present precarious food situation in very basic terms, reminding us that, as the population explosion brings millions more hungry mouths every year, we will in the future have little choice but to eat mostly vegetable food. Her book outlines the basis of such a sustaining diet. The amount of protein that can be taken from a given area of land is far greater when it is vegetable protein than when it is protein from animal sources, such as beef, poultry, lamb or pork.

Pork and poultry also appear in the Chinese diet. These animals are scavengers which do not have to subsist on the same foods which man might eat. The Chinese use a lot of fish in their cuisine. These take up no space on land. From ancient times Chinese farmers have stocked fish in their irrigation pools and harvested them in autumn when the water was no longer needed in the fields. Ducks and geese are also popular items in the Chinese diet. Although mutton and beef have been eaten, it is only in small quantities.

Traditionally, the Chinese attained the reputation of being the world's best, most adaptable and thrifty farmers. Partly by following tradition, partly through close association with their land, they developed masterpieces of irrigation and planting practices which allow them to use land that might be considered marginal in other localities. They may plant as many as three crops in the same field at the same time, each ripening at a different time.

The Chinese have grown, over the centuries, a wide variety of foods. They specialize in vegetables, including ones that appear exotic to us, like the lotus root and the water chestnut. They grow grapefruit (pomelos), oranges, bananas, pineapples, pawpaws (papaya), pears, cherries, peaches, apricots, walnuts, lichee nuts (*Litchi Chinensis*), chestnuts, grapes, plums and apples in different parts of the country, depending on climate. Bamboo shoots provide food, while the rest of the plant is used for countless other purposes.

With the exception of fish, complete protein is scarce in such a diet. The protein of the ancient Chinese was supplied largely by grain and legumes. In the South, rice is the chief cereal and is still eaten at every meal. Thousands of varieties of rice have been developed for use in China, almost all of them belonging to the botanical genus *Oryza,* species *sativa.* Chinese documents which are at least 5,000 years old show that, at that time, the right to sow rice was reserved for the emperor or some of his staff. So we know that rice was being cultivated in China as early as 5,000 years ago. Rice, alone among cereals, must grow part of the time in water, so rice fields must be flooded to a depth of several feet.

After the rice has flowered, the water is drained off to encourage the plant to build up its seeds at the expense of stem, leaves and root. The foliage withers and the crop is cut by hand. Threshing of rice is still done in a primitive way in many Far Eastern countries. World production of rice at present is about 300 million tons a year, of which China produces about one-third.

In some parts of China rice is almost unknown, while wheat, sorghum and millet form the cereal base of the diet. Barley, buckwheat and oats are staples in other parts of this vast country. Legumes have also been grown by the Chinese for thousands of years. Legumes like peas, alfalfa, clover and beans, including soybeans, are crops which enrich the soil while they are growing, so they should be an important part of any good farmer's plantings.

For many centuries the Chinese have made the soybean a source for many products: oil, soy sauce, bean curd, soup, and other traditional foods. They use soy oil cake for fertilizer and for feeding hogs. Soybeans have been raised in China for more than 4,000 years and have provided the main source of protein for all those generations of Chinese.

The soybean is the richest source of nearly complete protein in the vegetable kingdom. The immature seeds are almost 10 percent protein. Mature, dried and cooked, they contain 11 percent protein, while cooked rice is only 2½ percent protein. Other soy products are also rich in nearly complete protein. *Natto* is 17 percent protein and *miso* (cereal and soybeans) is 10½ percent protein. Soybean curd (the cheese of the Chinese) is almost 8 percent protein.

Peanuts and sweet potatoes have long been staple Chinese foods. Rape (*Brassica Napus*) is raised for its seeds which ripen before those of rice and cotton, for its new shoots which become salad greens, and for its dried stems which are burned for fuel. Sesame seed is another traditional Chinese crop, valued chiefly as a source of oil which does not easily become rancid.

Reay Tannahill tells us in *Food and History* how bean curd and soy sauce were traditionally made in China. Soybeans are simmered to a puree and the "milk" is drained off. This is boiled and the sediment which forms is dried to make bean curd. The puree is made into loaves and stored over the winter to ferment. Then the fungoid coating which develops is scraped off and the loaves are soaked in brine for a few weeks. The salty liquid which results is soy sauce. It is very salty, with 7,325 milligrams of sodium for every 100 grams—not a food to be used as a salt substitute by someone whose doctor has advised a low salt diet. What remains of the loaves is made into a thick cheese.

From earliest days the Chinese have sprouted soybeans, as well as other kinds of beans and peas, by leaving them, slightly damp, in a dark place until the sprouts form. Bean sprouts, rich in vitamin C and the B vitamins, are familiar ingredients in Chinese dishes today.

The ancient Chinese who were rich had a varied and delicious diet. A third century poem describes a meal of rice, broom corn, early wheat, yellow millet, ox-ribs, stewed turtle, roast kid with yam sauce, geese in sour sauce, duck, crane, braised chickens, fried honey cakes made of rice flour, sugar-malt sweetmeats and wine. The classic five flavors (bitter, sweet, salt, sour and hot) were the basis of Chinese flavoring and probably one of the reasons for the fine reputation of Chinese cooking.

It was probably the Chinese peasant who introduced the single most characteristic feature of Chinese cooking— the stir-fry technique. From early spring until the harvest was in, the Chinese peasant or farmer moved to temporary huts in the field. Fuel, always in short supply in China, was nearly impossible for him to find, so cooking had to be done in the shortest possible time. Rice, which required boiling, could be brought from home and eaten cold or re-heated. But meat, fish and vegetables were sliced as finely as possible and stirred briefly in a pot over a fire, so that they cooked in a few moments. Very thin pancakes of wheat or millet could be cooked the same way. Poor peasants used almost any food that could be found, including "brushwood eels" (snakes), "brushwood shrimp" (grasshoppers), and "household deer" (rats).

From early times the Chinese have been known as people who eat their meat or fish raw or almost raw. Lack of fuel must have been the reason, as it was with primitive Eskimos. Learned doctors used to protest against this practice, for there are dangers to health in raw fish and raw meat, especially pork. Marco Polo used the word "Tartar" for the Chinese, so it seems likely that the name of our "Steak Tartar" comes from his descriptions of ancient Chinese eating raw meat.

A classic example of the harm we do by refining food is the story of white rice and beriberi. Rice is the staple food of millions of Oriental people. It is a fairly adequate staple food. If eaten in quantity it supplies enough protein to serve as the protein base of a national diet, along with other complementary sources of vegetable protein.

Unfortunately, the Oriental people found that they could polish rice, removing the outer coating to make a fine, white, shiny rice berry which they preferred to brown or unrefined rice. So white rice became the basic food in many parts of the East. Very soon thereafter a disease appeared which all but wiped out large areas of that part of the world.

The disease was beriberi. As late as the end of World War I, a survey in the Philippines showed that nearly 13 percent of the population had beriberi. The annual mortality was 132 out of every 100,000 people. One fifth of all disease in Malaya was attributed to beriberi. In the Philippines it was second only to tuberculosis as a cause of death. Between 1920 and 1929 there were 17,000 deaths annually from beriberi in Japan.

It took a long time for scientists to discover the cause of beriberi. But finally the evidence was irrefutable. It is caused simply by lack of the various vitamins and minerals which are removed when rice is polished. It is cured by re-placing those nutrients in the diet. Chiefly it is a disease of thiamine (vitamin B1) deficiency, but also involved are the other vitamins and minerals in the rice coating. Beriberi does not appear in countries where a widely varied diet is eaten even when white rice is a staple food. The other foods provide the missing vitamins and minerals.

But when white rice is just about the only food eaten day after day, there is just no way to avoid beriberi. This terrible disease involves nervous and circulatory troubles, fatigue, cramps in the legs, paralysis, irritability, lack of appetite, headache, fast heart beat, loss of sight, edema and many other disabling symptoms. Thiamine is injected as an emergency treatment. But the diet must be corrected to contain plenty of thiamine, as well as all the other vitamins and minerals found in unrefined cereals.

The Chinese national beverage is, of course, tea. It is known botanically as *Camellia sinensis*. Many thousands of years ago, tribesmen in Southern China discovered that dried tea leaves, put into hot water, produce a pleasant taste and a stimulating effect on the body. The stimulant is an alkaloid *theine* which acts like the caffeine in coffee. Tea also contains smaller amounts of caffeine.

Nowadays there are many varieties of tea and the method of curing determines what kind of tea the finished product will be. Black or Indian tea is fermented for about 36 hours to develop its distinctive taste. Chinese tea is steamed but not allowed to ferment, so it retains its green color. Oolong tea is partially fermented. All teas are dried quickly over low heat. Tea was originally grown only in China and neighboring countries. It was carried overland on camel trains across the Gobi Desert to Europe. Later the "clipper ships" brought tea around the Cape of Good Hope to Britain and America.

The diet of the Chinese is traditionally short on calcium, since the best sources of this mineral are milk and milk products. The use of white rice rather than brown rice leads to deficiencies in other vitamins and minerals which must be made up by other foods at daily meals. To get enough protein, the rice-eating inhabitant of the Far East must eat large amounts of rice, for the average 3½ ounce serving contains only about two grams of protein. So protein-rich soybeans and peanuts are essential foods for rice-eating countries.

One reason why the Chinese diet has remained adequate to sustain this large nation down through thousands of years, in spite of floods and droughts, is undoubtedly the care the farmers give their land. No natural fertility, even as great as that of some of China's alluvial plains, could have yielded, unassisted, such continuous returns over so long a time as has the soil of China without the continued persistence and skill of the Chinese farmer who keeps his fields well supplied with compost and natural fertilizers.

Growing legumes which provide nitrogen to the soil

97

is only one of China's agricultural skills. The Chinese also return everything organic to the soil, in the best organic gardening tradition. Compost piles have always been familiar sights in the Chinese landscape. Human waste is also composted, to remove harmful organisms, and then returned to the soil, rather than being flushed away to contaminate water supplies as we do in the West. All animal manure is carefully used as fertilizer. Ashes, containing precious minerals, are scattered over the land. Soil from canals containing silt is returned to the fields. Crops are rotated—all in the best tradition of what we know is good agricultural practice.

At the very opposite dietetic extreme from the milk-hating, near-vegetarian Chinese, were the Kazakhs of what is now Soviet Asia. They lived almost entirely on milk and milk products and enjoyed good health. Their society flourished for thousands of years on such a diet.

The Kazakhs who presently live in the Kazakh Soviet Republic, are descended from these nomadic people who, for thousands of years, herded their cattle, goats, sheep, camels and horses over the vast plains and into the mountains of Central Asia. Moving almost constantly from place to place to provide fodder for their animals, they could not plant grain, trees or vegetable gardens. They lived, almost completely, on the products of their animals. Since they ate comparatively little meat in summer, to spare their animals, their diet consisted almost entirely of milk products.

The Kazakh home was a *yurt,* a convenient collapsible tent which they carried with them. All cooking was done on an open fire built in the middle of the *yurt.* In spring they migrated to fresh pastures, carrying all their belongings with them.

They knew many ways of preparing milk and cheese. There was *koumiss,* fermented mare's milk which was served on special occasions. *Koumiss* was made as we make yogurt today. A little "starter" saved from the last batch of *koumiss* was added to fresh warm milk.

Helen and George Papashvily tell us in *Russian Cooking* that the *koumiss* was then hung in a bag of smoked horseskin for 24 hours. Then fresh mare's milk was added and the preparation was churned for an hour, after which the milk was left to ferment, then churned again. After a third period of fermentation and beating, the *koumiss* was tasted to see if it had enough alcoholic content. "A bag of the finished brew often hung outside the *yurt* for hospitable refreshment and proper etiquette required that anyone who passed within arm's length should agitate the bag just to keep the *koumiss* shaken up," say the Papashvilys.

Kazakhs also made a hard cheese called *kurt* which was shaped into a hard sphere and stored. It kept for a long time. In winter *kurt* was grated, mixed with water and drunk in place of milk. There was also a kind of soft cheese like our cottage cheese.

George Murdock in *Our Primitive Contemporaries* tells us that in summer rich Kazakhs subsisted almost entirely on *koumiss,* drinking it in enormous quantities. Since it is only mildly intoxicating (one to two percent alcohol), we assume they did not thereby court alcoholism. In autumn, the Kazakhs slaughtered some sheep and goats which they could not manage to feed all winter. At this time they ate large quantities of meat, two to four pounds a day, with no ill effects. The fat tail of the sheep was considered a special delicacy.

Murdock says that a Kazakh migration was a festive sight. The women were dressed in their brightest clothing, with red saddlecloths on their horses. Children were carried in their cradles on red sacks over the pommels of the saddles. Men and children, mounted on goats, ponies, horses, with pack animals laden with belongings and herds of animals

99

kept in line by shepherds and dogs, stretched sometimes for several miles.

The staple, almost the only food, of the Kazakhs was milk. Milk is notoriously short on iron. Where did the old-time Kazakhs get their iron? Obviously people leading such a vigorous life are not suffering from widespread anemia.

The Papashvilys speculate that perhaps the deep wells from which they got their water gave the nomads ample iron. During their stay in the Kazakh Republic the Papash-vilys met an ancient lady near Alma Ata who told them she remembered when her people were nomads. She could tell, she said, from only one mouthful of *koumiss,* which mare had given the milk. All the mares had names. She could not tell from which ewe the sheep milk came, since ewes were not named.

But, she said, "I could tell how the ewe was fed and what flowers had bloomed where she pastured and the age of her lamb . . . by tasting sheep's milk my grandmother could tell whether the ewe had borne a male or female, but my grandmother's tongue was better than most peoples' ears and nose together. One time, when she was still living in her father's *yurt,* a servant driving part of their flock to pasture sent back word that a certain sheep had borne a single lamb. But when the milk was brought in, my grandmother tasted *twin* lambs—and so it proved to be. The servant had intended to keep that extra lamb for himself."

These days milk comes to us in plastic containers. It is the product of a large number of dairy farms which pool their milk. The feed for dairy cattle is a standardized mix. A standardized fertilizer is used on fields on which the food is grown. Isn't it possible that, in the times when the Kazakhs roamed the plains, their animals, grazing, sought out the most mineral-rich plants that grew? So perhaps their milk was indeed not lacking in iron or any trace mineral

100

essential for the proper use of iron by the body. There is no way to check this. We cannot return to those ancient days and do laboratory tests on the grasses and flowers eaten by individual mares and ewes. But there is every possibility that the animals may have had far more innate sense about these things than we give them credit for. If indeed the ancient Alma Ata woman could tell which mare gave which pint of milk, there must have been great variations in the pasture available for the animals.

What about vitamin C? There's enough vitamin C in fresh milk, so the Kazakhs would not have suffered from scurvy in spring, summer and autumn. But what about winter when they had almost nothing to eat but cheese and some meat? Is it possible that enough vitamin C remained in this hard, dry cheese to sustain them through the winter? We are not told of cases of scurvy among them. Possibly scurvy did exist. Possibly, too, their way of preparing the cheese somehow preserved the vitamin C so that they were never short on this essential vitamin.

Another question which would certainly be asked by the cholesterol-conscious element of our nutrition establishment is how did the Kazakhs survive without heart and artery conditions thinning their ranks, when they must have consumed enormous amounts of cholesterol every day? They were a hardy lot. There is no record of their population being thinned by plagues like hardening of the arteries and heart attacks.

Part of the reason, as it seems to be with the present-day Masai and related nations in Africa, must have been the daily exercise they got. Many scientists today believe that our sedentary lives are at least partly responsible for our circulatory troubles. Another group of scientists has presented some formidable evidence in support of another theory—that of refined carbohydrates being largely responsible for heart attacks and hardening of the arteries.

The ancient Kazakhs did not use any form of sugar. They did not even have access to honey. They used no grains, no vegetables. Their entire carbohydrate intake was the lactose (sugar) found in milk. Everything else in their diet was protein and fat. And for thousands of years they dominated the plains of Central Asia, living out of doors, in unpolluted air, drinking unpolluted water and eating unpolluted food. These latter considerations must partly explain their rollicking good health.

From Miguel Covarrubias' book, *Island of Bali,* we get some idea of food the Balinese ate when he visited them in the 1930's. Rice was prepared by boiling it in a clay pot or, more elaborately, by washing the rice repeatedly until the water lost its milky color and came out transparent (probably washing away a great deal of the nutriment, unfortunately, since this lies close to the outer skin). The rice was then boiled. When half-cooked, it was put into a funnel-shaped basket and steamed over boiling water. Some of the water was scooped over the rice to keep it from sticking together. Rice served as the basis for extremely hot sauces made of coconut and chili peppers.

Although the food was frugal, says Covarrubias, the Balinese seemed exceptionally well-fed. They were always nibbling at something. They snacked at odd hours, buying foods at public eating booths, at the market, at crossroads and especially at festivals where they ate peanuts and drank many local beverages. Street vendors sold roast chicken with a package of cooked rice for six cents. The orders were wrapped in neat little packages of banana leaves.

Snacking five or six times a day rather than eating just one, two or three large meals has been recommended by many modern nutrition experts. Undoubtedly this was the way our earliest ancestors ate, since they ate whatever they happened to find in their food-gathering travels.

Food is always served cold in Bali, says Covarrubias, and to make it tastier it is always accompanied by crushed roots and leaves, nuts, onions, garlic, fermented fish paste, lemon juice, grated coconut and "burning red peppers . . . so hot that it made even me, a Mexican raised on chili peppers, cry and break out in beads of perspiration." Babies are fed the hot, peppery foods from infancy, he tells us, and in adult life they will not touch food without spices and peppers in it. They find European food tasteless.

In general, Covarrubias explains, the Balinese eat everything that walks, swims, flies or crawls. At the time he was there they were not permitted by their religion to eat tigers, monkeys, dogs, crocodiles, mice, snakes, frogs, certain poisonous fish, leeches, stinging insects, crows, eagles, owls and in general "all birds with moustaches." They ate pork, chicken, duck, beef, buffalo, dragonflies, crickets, flying ants and the larvae of bees.

Boys catch dragonflies on long poles smeared with a sticky sap. The wings are removed and the bodies are fried in coconut oil with spices and vegetables. The Balinese hunt and eat anteaters, flying fox (which is their name for a fruit-eating bat), porcupines, lizards, wild boar, squid, many kinds of birds, crayfish and fried eels.

There are many vegetable foods: rice, corn, sweet potatoes, eggplant, papaya, coconut, bananas, pineapples, mangoes, melons, oranges, peanuts, breadfruit, jackfruit (another kind of breadfruit), greens, edible ferns, a pear-shaped fruit that grows on a palm—"tastes like a pineapple and is covered by the most perfect imitation snakeskin," the *rambutan* —a large sort of grape inside of a hairy transparent pink skin, and the mangosteen. Our horticultural encyclopedia defines this as "one of the most luscious of tropical fruits, produced by an evergreen tree, *Garcinia Mangostana.*" Queen

Victoria offered a prize to anyone who could manage to bring some of this superlative fruit, in good condition, to England.

Then there is the *durian* (*Durio zibethinus*). Covarrubias describes this spiky custard apple "whose putrid smell has been compared with every decaying or evil-smelling thing from goats to rancid butter." Most Europeans forbid their servants to bring *durian* within a distance of their house.

But the fruit is apparently blissfully delicious when you eat it. Says Dr. Enlin in *Plants and Man,* "The *durian* ripens at the top of a tall jungle tree and then falls to the ground. Pigs, monkeys, bears and even tigers compete with man to eat the fallen fruits. Malays build temporary shelters close to the trees so as to be on the spot when the great *durians* come hurtling down." The fruit is huge and contains many seeds which are about the size of a chestnut.

Covarrubias says that the Balinese make a delicious dessert of coconut cream with cinnamon, bananas or breadfruit steamed in packages of banana leaf.

For a Balinese festival, which Covarrubias attended, the men did most of the cooking. They prepared a huge turtle, whose blood they had collected and spiked with lime juice to keep it from coagulating. (Could it be the vitamin C which does this?) There are many traditional Balinese ways of serving turtle meat: chopped with spices and raw blood, chopped with coconut and spices, first chopped with coconut and spices, then mixed with coconut cream or cooked in tamarind leaves. Turtle meat paste is made by pounding and chopping the meat, then kneading into it spices and coconuts. The whole thing is put on a bamboo spit and roasted over a fire.

The traditional sauce boggles the mind, or perhaps one should say the taste-buds. Red pepper, garlic and red onions are first sauteed, then mixed with black pepper, ginger, turmeric, nutmeg, cloves, *srá* (fermented fish paste) and some roots like ginger. Salt is added and the toasted skin of a coconut. This mixture is then fried in coconut oil, a whole grated coconut is added, and the dough that remains is kneaded for as long as an hour and a half. Then the dough is carefully put on the spit and roasted over the coals. This dish is called *saté*. It can be served with pork, chicken or duck as well as turtle.

Suckling pigs are stuffed with a sauce like the one described above and the skin of the pig is rubbed with turmeric mixed with water. It is impaled on a bamboo stick and roasted over the fire for several hours. This is called *beguling*. It is unsurpassed in flavor and texture, according to Covarrubias.

With either or both of these main dishes, the Balinese always serve rice, along with many chopped mixtures of *satés:* fried beans, bean sprouts with crushed peanuts, parched grated coconut or preserved salted eggs. And they drink a palm beer or *brom,* a sweet sherry made from fermented black rice, or *arak,* a distilled rice brandy. They did not drink to become intoxicated, says Covarrubias. He says he never saw a drunken Balinese in all the time he spent there.

Chapter
8

Some African Peoples
Have Great Abundance,
Others Eat Sparingly

We get most of our information about the food of ancient Egyptians from tombs where lists of food offerings and sometimes remnants of foods themselves have been found. Ancient Egyptians had many kinds of breads and cakes. Shapes and sizes varied. The *shat* cake, for example, took the shape of an isosceles triangle. Another Egyptian bread was made in conical shape. The baker heated an earthenware baking mold until it was very hot, then lined the inside with a layer of dough. The heat held by the mold baked the dough right there. No need to put it in an oven.

Nine varieties of meat were mentioned in Egyptian tombs, including kidneys, two kinds of goose, also duck, teal and pigeons, and two kinds of cheese or possibly soured milk. Available vegetables included: onions, pumpkins, cucumbers, legumes, lettuce, and leeks. Fruits were pomegranates, grapes, many varieties of dates and the fruit of the *baobab* tree, called monkey bread because of wild monkeys' fondness for it.

Dessert was likely to be figs, melons or dates. Beverages were water and several kinds of beer and wine. Poor people ate mostly bread and onions with some cheese and fish, and drank only water.

Rich Egyptians probably ate well. Tombs contain varied foods which were to last them into the next world: barley, porridge, quail, fish, beef, wheat bread, cakes, stewed figs, fresh berries, cheese, wine and beer. Fish from the Nile were a popular food, eaten either fresh or dried and salted. Small birds were sometimes pickled and eaten raw.

The Egyptians probably discovered the use of yeast to raise bread. Some unknown Egyptian baker must have forgotten his bread dough and a yeasty organism from the air drifted into it. When the baker returned, he found the dough light and the bread tastier than the unleavened kind. It was only a matter of time until the Egyptians discovered that the mysterious substance which created this delicious bread was yeast—a ferment, as they called it.

There are still what we would call "primitive" people in Africa, living much as their forefathers lived, and eating the traditional foods. They are hard pressed to give up the old ways, for "progress" is surrounding them. Government officials of the new African nations want to industrialize their countries as quickly as possible, so they can compete with Western nations and share in the comforts and glories of Western opulence and culture.

One of the ancient primitive groups among Africans, closely studied because of their diet, is the Masai people. They are remarkable for their almost complete freedom from "civilized" diseases, including heart and circulatory disorders. They depend on their cattle for food. Throughout past centuries they have lived on milk, meat and blood, with a few vegetables and fruits. They milk their cows daily and bleed the steers at regular intervals by a special process. The blood is whipped to solidify the fibrin part which is then fried or cooked much as we cook bacon. The liquid part is used as a beverage. They judge the excellence of their cattle not by the amount of milk they produce, which is our main criterion, but by the health of their calves. A calf which can leap up and run, only moments after birth, is thought to be superior.

No one knows why we deposit the fatty substance cholesterol on the inner walls of our arteries. Nor does anyone know why some people have these troublesome accumulations and others do not. We have been told that our sedentary lives have something to do with our national proclivity to hardening of the arteries caused, many scientists believe, by cholesterol deposits. Some segments of the medical establishment claim it is the amount of fatty food we eat and the relative proportions of fat from animal sources and fat from vegetable sources. We have also been told that stress has something to do with it—and smoking.

Two Illinois researchers reported in *The New York Times,* September 12, 1968, on a study they made of the Masai, who are, incidentally, tall, graceful, slim and beautifully built—all of them. Obesity is unknown and heart disease is rare. Yet, since these people live almost entirely on blood, meat and milk, almost every mouthful of food contains cholesterol. Their daily diets contain at least as much of this fatty substance as does "the average American diet." How does it happen, then, that the cholesterol eaten by the Masai does not go awry in their bodies to become a threat to life, as it does in the bodies of many Americans?

The two scientists, Dr. C. Bruce Taylor and Dr. Kangjey Ho, tried an experiment with two groups of Masai. Both groups ate their usual fatty diet, but the two scientists fed additional pure cholesterol to one of the groups. At the end of the experiment, the two groups were found to have exactly the same levels of cholesterol in their blood. Giving a similar group of Americans such a test, say the researchers, would show that the more cholesterol eaten, the higher the level of this fat would be in the blood.

Why this difference? The Illinois scientists believe there is something quite different about the way the livers and intestines of the Masai people handle fatty substances, compared with the way these mechanisms operate in most Americans. Perhaps the tendency is inherited, they surmise. And perhaps some Americans have the same ability to eat plenty of cholesterol-rich food and suffer no harm from it, due to the same hereditary mechanism. After they finish their studies, the scientists hope to evolve a test which could be applied to individual Americans, early in life, to determine whether they are inherently susceptible to cholesterol deposits. If so, the doctors propose, the individual could alter his diet or take cholesterol-reducing drugs to remain healthy.

The most obvious fault with these investigations is that they don't go far enough. Why not investigate and compare *everything* about the Masai diet and the American diet—not just the cholesterol content? The Masai eat no carbohydrate foods at all, except for a few roots or berries. Certainly they eat no refined carbohydrates—those white sugar and white flour products which make up about half the average diet in Western countries. Many competent nutrition experts believe our diets have become completely unbalanced by this heavy load of carbohydrates, especially since they enter our bodies with almost none of the vitamins and minerals that accompany carbohydrates in wholly natural foods such as fruits, vegetables and whole-grain cereals.

If the Masai could be persuaded to engage in a more conclusive far-reaching test, they could be given "the average American diet" with its load of white bread, cakes, soft drinks, candy, coffee, alcohol and pastries, to see what such a diet would do to cholesterol levels and heart health. Their body mechanisms might then become so disordered that the Masai, too, might begin to store cholesterol in arteries and might become susceptible to all the circulatory troubles that afflict so many Western people.

In the *Journal of the American Medical Association* for April 23, 1973, we are told that the story of the Bedouins is almost a perfect example of such a test. These nomads have lived in the desert for centuries on almost nothing but the meat and milk products from their herds. In the past 14 or 15 years many Bedouins have moved into cities. Heart attacks are becoming common among these people who have never before suffered from such disabilities.

Says the *Journal*, "The increasing incidence of coronary disease among Bedouins follows a familiar pattern. Recent immigrants from Yemen to Israel have a much lower rate of coronary disease than their comfortably settled relatives of comparable age. Similar observations have been made in immigrants from other underdeveloped areas. It would appear that those who live on the fringes of civilization must give up some fringe benefits when they embrace the good life."

The Bedouins have traditionally lived on diets extremely high in fat. City living offers them the delights of refined carbohydrates, as well as a supposedly easier life. The fat content in the Yemenite diets did not increase when they moved to Israel. But the sugar content increased greatly. And the circulatory diseases as well.

The Karimojong are a nation in Northeastern Uganda who, like the Masai, herd cattle and depend mostly on the milk and blood of their herds, along with some cereal food. An account of their lives appeared in *Scientific American* for February, 1969. According to the authors, Rada and Neville Dyson-Hudson, Westerners tend to think that the herding way of life of these primitive people is very irrational, and that they should be taught better and more economical methods of survival. But we just don't understand the complexities of the situation, the Dyson-Hudsons believe.

True, Karimojong life is chancy and insecure. The country is arid. There is no way of knowing where it will rain, how much, or how often. Karimojong men herd their cattle wherever there is good grazing. Women and children stay behind in a camp where they plant the one cereal food, sorghum. This way of doing things makes the most of the available resources.

While they are herding the cattle, the men live on milk and, from time to time, blood which they draw painlessly from the cattle. The women live mostly on the cereal they raise and, when the herds are near, they also have milk. When an animal dies or must be slaughtered because of drought, Karimojong culture demands that the meat be shared with relatives and friends. The immediate family benefits little from what might otherwise be a windfall. So cattle are more valued for their milk than for meat.

There are many more cattle than people. As few as 30 people may depend for their food on a herd of 200 cattle. Only about 12 percent of the cattle give milk. Many are male and cows do not become fresh until they are three and a half to four years old. There is a period of 14 months between calves, then a short lactation period of less than eight months. About half the cows give only enough milk to sustain their calves. Others give not much more than two pints a day beyond the needs of their calves in a dry season, or up to four pints a day in a good rainy season.

Karimojong men drink about two and a half pints of milk or more each day, along with blood. Women and children use about one pint of milk daily, along with whatever cereal they eat. Some of the milk is made into buttermilk and butter (in the form of *ghee*) since these foods keep better in the hot climate. Fruit of the tamarind, mushrooms, wild honey and some herbs make up the rest of the diet of this nation of 60,000 people.

No wonder agronomists grow impatient with such primitive arrangements and plan ambitious changes to butcher all surplus males and develop cows into milk factories as we Westerners have done with our cows. Instead of trailing around from place to place following the rains, there should be irrigation projects, fields planted to high yielding fodder and all the other essentials of a modern Western dairy farm. But the Karimojong have followed their present way of life for thousands of years. Their cattle are the very center of their universe. They are the dowry of new wives. Female animals are highly valued, never sold or killed. Young boys are given young male calves with which to identify, to care for and decorate.

There seems little doubt that, as civilization and industrialization proceed in Africa, the Karimojong will be forced to change their living habits. They have traditionally roamed over 4,000 square miles with complete freedom. As population pressures mount in Africa, such a way of life appears to be doomed. Yet Uganda scientists believe that measures to ameliorate the situation should be introduced only after very careful thought. The cattle-centered way of life of the Karimojong is closely tied up with their system of values and their culture. Their living, although precarious, is really a time-tested way of extracting a maximum amount of sustenance from a harsh, unpredictable terrain. The tragic widespread drought in parts of Africa which has prevailed now for more than five years may finally wipe out cattle-centered nations like that of the Karimojong and the Masai. Whatever small remnants of such societies survive the current drought disaster will almost certainly have to rely on some other means of livelihood, if only because so many of their cattle have died.

What happened to another African nation, the Ik, when they were abruptly uprooted from their traditional way of life and forced into another, is told with agonizing detail in a recent book, *The Mountain People,* by Colin M. Turnbull. The Ik, who live north of the Karimojong, were a hunting people for as long as they existed. Their land was made into a national park in an effort to preserve some of Africa's fast disappearing, irreplaceable wildlife. Hunting became illegal.

For generations the men of the Ik had hunted coopera-tively, with bows and arrows, spears or nets. They considered it a major crime to overhunt. They took only what they needed to sustain them that day. Women and children, mean-while, gathered whatever other food was available in the way of roots, berries, leaves, honey or insects.

Hunters in a hunting society must, of necessity, develop such character traits as kindness, generosity, consideration, affection, honesty, compassion and charity, says Turnbull, for they depend for their survival on the friends and relatives who help them hunt.

When the Ik were removed from their hunting land, they were told to plant gardens and cereal crops. But with no equipment, no knowledge of such a way of getting food, and no interest in it, the Ik became, within one generation, "as unfriendly, as uncharitable, inhospitable, and generally mean as any people can be," says Turnbull. The much more basic man who developed under these circumstances had no time for friendliness or generosity. Faced with day-by-day starvation every individual had to become concerned only with his own welfare.

The Ik were starving to death during the time that Turnbull lived with them and studied them. One by one, they simply dropped and died and no one bothered to bury them. For, by now, Ik culture had completely disintegrated. None of the old ways were left. People fought for food. They had, seemingly, no meaningful relationships left

114

among them. Hunger was the only concern of every day. Children were thrust out of the home at the age of three to fend for themselves. Old people were totally neglected and laughed at. If a child or a feeble old person managed to find a tidbit of food, it was snatched from them by almost anyone strong enough to do it. And the thief laughed at the despair of his starving son or grandfather.

Ashley Montagu said of this book, "The parallel with our own society is deadly. If we would see ourselves for what we have become we would do well to read it."

What we learn from *The Mountain People* is that you dare not suddenly disrupt a long established culture, especially with regard to food and traditional ways of obtaining it, and expect that culture to survive. Over a long period of time, permitted to ease gradually into an agricultural way of life, perhaps the Ik could have made it. But they were *suddenly* forbidden to hunt. They were *suddenly* moved from their hunting grounds. And, in one generation, they became dehumanized and their long-established culture disintegrated.

Dr. Samuel Rosen, a famous ear specialist, travelled widely in Africa a few years ago to test the hearing of African people still living in the bush. His most astonishing discovery was the Mabaans, who, according to an article in *Parade* for September 1, 1963, have a life that is anything but easy.

Their diet consists mostly of a sour, pasty bread called *durrah*. The climate shifts between two seasons—blistering heat and pelting rainstorms. But Dr. Rosen found the Mabaans to be tall, muscular people who remain surprisingly healthy into a very old age. "They do not die until their bodies completely wear out," he said. Which means, of course, that they do not suffer from the diseases of civilization.

Most surprising of all, Dr. Rosen found that the hearing of the Mabaans is so acute they can hear a soft murmur across a distance the length of a football field. They have the best hearing of any of the people he tested and it does not degenerate with age. Nor does their blood pressure rise with age. There are no heart attacks among the Mabaans. Is the reason their diet, which is almost fat-free? Dr. Rosen thinks not, for a neighboring tribe, the Samburu, eat a diet consisting of 65 percent fat and they, too, have no heart disease and live to a great age, in very good health.

Dr. Rosen believes the answer may lie in the kind of life they lead: absence of noise, a peaceful life, no pressures. At any rate, it seems certain that a high fat diet cannot possibly be the one and only cause of circulatory disorders.

It should not surprise you to discover that, when the Mabaans move into town (Khartoum, the nearest "civilized" point) they, too, begin very soon to succumb to "civilized" diseases—heart attacks, strokes, ulcers and all the rest.

Dr. T. L. Cleave and Dr. G. D. Campbell have extensively documented the very same conditions with regard to other African groups who leave their ancestral homes and diets and migrate to cities, where they exist on Western food. Their very convincing books on this subject are listed in the bibliography.

In *African Cooking,* Laurens Van der Post describes food in modern Ethiopia which derives from ancient ways of eating. He details one meal at which he was served raw meat, moist and still warm. Each diner took the edge of the meat between his teeth, then sliced off a bit, barely missing his nose. The meat was then dipped into a hot sauce called *berberé,* which is widely used. It is full of powdered pepper with many spices and herbs. Van der Post says the sauce gives the impression of being hot enough to cook the raw meat.

116

Berberé also appears in stews and in the national dish called *wat.* There are chicken *wats* and vegetable *wats* for vegetarians. The chicken dish might contain powdered ginger, ground black pepper, powdered cardamom, minced onion, lemon juice, hard boiled eggs and chicken. The vegetable *wat* might have diced peas, lentils, chick-peas, beans, onions and fresh ginger.

Many other herbs and spices are used in Ethiopia: fenugreek, coriander, cumin, fennel seed, red pepper, garlic, basil, bishop's weed (*Aegopodium*—we call it goutweed), rue, mint, cloves, cinnamon, turmeric and nutmeg.

Ethiopians eat without utensils. They dip their bread— usually like a thick pancake—into the main dish with the right hand and soak up the liquids or wrap a solid ingredient such as a piece of meat, in the bread, to eat it.

They have many kinds of bread made of wheat, millet or barley. To make *teff,* a bread of finely ground millet, they mix the flour with water, then allow the batter to ferment for three or four days, then pour the batter on a flat clay griddle and cook for about five minutes to make a fine, bubbly pancake.

A farmer in West Africa lives on milk, curds, whey, green vegetables, peas, beans, cereals, cassava, and seeds from the *baobab* tree which are crushed and ground to flavor foods. Also sweet potatoes and yams, many wild fruits and leaves.

Yams (not the same thing as sweet potatoes, remember) are the basis of the diet. Feast days are celebrated in honor of yams. To prepare yams the Africans boil, then peel, slice or pound them to a paste which is called *fufu.* This may be made into a croquette and fried in palm or peanut oil. It may be flattened and deep-fried into a kind of potato chip. It may be cooked with palm nuts, boiled in milk or used in ragouts or stews. Modern Africans also use *fufu*

117

finely sliced with onions, grated cheese and breadcrumbs in casseroles.

The banana and its close relative, the plantain, are widely used in West Africa. Almost any kind of dish can be made of these versatile fruits: croquettes, purees served with eggs, banana custards or wine. Peanuts with their high protein content are also an important food. They are pounded and made into sauce for shrimps or prawns. They are used in chicken dishes with tomatoes, onions, peppers and garlic. This might be served with rice, *fufu,* hard-boiled eggs, eggplant, fried plantains, pineapple with diced papaya and grated coconut.

Many dishes have a coconut base. Chickens are roasted with a sauce made from coconuts cooked in their own milk. Coconut oil is cooked with rice. African chicken is generally tough, so it is usually cut up and pounded to tenderize it, or wrapped in pawpaw (*papaya*) leaves to tenderize it. Papaya contains an enzyme which tenderizes meat. This enzyme is the basis for our American meat tenderizers.

When Dr. Weston Price visited in Africa he found tribes in Eastern and Central Africa using large amounts of sweet potatoes, beans and cereals, plus fish and cattle where they were available. He was impressed with their use of insects as food. In Lake Victoria and other bodies of water, certain winged insects are hatched in vast numbers, so that they accumulate on the shore. The Africans gathered them, dried and preserved them for puddings.

Then, too, clever ways had been developed to capture the ants which build huge anthills ten feet or more in height. Africans living nearby know the time of mating season when the ants leave the nests in large numbers. The occasion is usually during or following a rain. So the Africans induce the ants to come out by covering the opening of the hills with leaves to give the effect of clouds and darkness, then pounding on the ground to imitate rainfall.

The vast swarms of locusts (various kinds of grass-hoppers) which plague African farmers are gathered in huge amounts, cooked for immediate use, or ground into flour for later use.

Dr. Price investigated what was in knapsacks in many parts of the world. In the Andes, in Central Africa and among the Aborigines of Australia, he found knapsacks to contain little balls of clay. When the native people ate, they often dissolved a bit of clay in water and dipped morsels of food into it. This, they said, was to prevent sick stomach. Dr. Price was later treated with a clay compound when he got dysentery in Central Africa. Modern medicine in our country uses clay in the form of *kaolin* to treat bacterial infections of the digestive tract.

There Are Many
Pacific Islands and Many
Delightful People Live There

The Price of Civilization is the title of an article which appeared in *Nutrition Today*, July/August, 1971. Its author, Ian A. M. Prior, M.D., is Director of the Epidemiology Unit at the Wellington Hospital in New Zealand. His article and the intriguing chart which accompanies it show comparative figures on diet and disease among four groups of South Seas people. The road to civilization is, it seems, made infinitely more dangerous and life-threatening by the diseases of civilization.

Dr. Prior and a distinguished staff of medical and para-medical personnel are studying the Polynesian residents of the South Seas in terms of three historical groups—those who have already succumbed to the "benefits" of civilization, those who are only partially "civilized" and those who are living almost as their ancestors have lived for thousands of years. The object of the study is to discover how diet and way of life influence the incidence of such diseases as obesity, high blood pressure, cholesterol levels, gout, diabetes, and ischemic heart disease, a condition that brings on heart attacks.

Dr. Prior says of the Polynesians that they are handsome, brave and intelligent. No one knows where they came

121

from or how long they have inhabited this part of the Pacific Ocean. They can be traced back to Tahiti, but not beyond that. The Maoris are believed to have migrated southwest across the ocean in their sea-faring canoes, leaving colonies along the way. Their last migration was to New Zealand, where they arrived in the 14th century.

Captain Cook found them well established there 400 years later and, as the white men began to colonize the islands, they conquered the Maoris with the expected bloodshed, finally making peace of a sort by 1871—about the same kind of peace we Americans have made with our Indian population.

The Maoris now make up about one-tenth of New Zealand's population of nearly three million. Their life expectancy is only 57 years, while that of the white New Zealander is 72 years. The New Zealand Maoris, by now well established in the white man's civilization, appear to be far more susceptible to high blood pressure, heart disease, diabetes, gout and related disorders than their relatives who still live on remote islands. Four to five times as many women living in New Zealand, both European and Maori, suffer from high blood pressure as those women who live on atolls far from "civilization."

Dr. Prior's group chose the South Pacific Island of Rarotonga as a place to study a people slowly emerging from primitive society into civilized society. The Island of Pukapuka was chosen as the island most suitable for a study of people still living mostly as their ancestors lived for thousands of years.

Dr. Prior's group included a cardiologist, a specialist in heart and respiratory diseases, a pediatrician, an anthropologist, a nutrition expert, a home economist and specialists in electrocardiography. Also included were many native Polynesians who were delighted to help in any way they could.

The name of the steamer on which they sailed to Pukapuka was *Akatere,* which means, in Maori, "go quickly". It took them six delightful, lazy days to go the 700 miles from Rarotonga to Pukapuka.

When they landed, the people greeted them warmly and hospitably, starting a round of festivities. Prior found them a "blissfully happy" lot, living in a completely un-sophisticated society with almost no knowledge of the myriad complex troubles that vex the rest of the world.

The scientists wanted to collect urine, since they would be studying the role of salt and other minerals in the local diet. The Pukapukans were pleased to cooperate. They proudly carried around the little flasks they were given wherever they went, contentedly contributing their share to the scientific fact-finding.

The nutritionists who analyzed food and urine found that these people eat almost no salt. Even the bread that was available had not been salted. The Pukapukans have indi-vidual annual incomes of about $36 in American money, but nothing much to buy with it. Boats call at the island three or four times a year to buy *copra,* the dried white flesh of coconuts, used for coconut oil.

Since there is no place to buy much Western food, the Pukapukans still live mostly on what their ancestors ate for thousands of years: fish, taro, cassava and coconuts in many forms, with "modest" supplements of rice, flour and sugar, and almost no salt. Flour and sugar are brought in by the *copra* boats infrequently. The Pukapukans have pigs and chickens.

Taro (Colocasia esculenta) is a tuberous root of which several hundred varieties are known. Polynesians use it to make their thin porridge called *poi. Taro* feeds millions of people in this part of the world. It was probably originally domesticated in southeastern Asia, our earliest record of it being in China. Eventually brought to Africa, it was taken to the United States by slaves who planted it in our South. It did not become popular there, since it was competing with many other root crops.

The *taro* plant looks like the "elephant's ear" we use as a house plant. It is related to our colorful caladiums and to the philodendron which every house-plant lover knows. Jack-in-the-pulpit is another well-known member of the family. The roots contain a bitter substance—oxalic acid crystals which can be toxic. Like many other plant poisons, they are rendered harmless by boiling. Taro roots are about 30 percent starch, three percent sugar and only about two percent protein, which is not very much. They are good sources of potassium. The leaves contain much more protein than the roots, as well as large amounts of vitamin A, vitamin C and the B vitamins.

To make *poi* out of *taro,* the Polynesians steam the roots, crush them, make them into a thin dough and ferment the dough for several days. They eat *poi* by dipping in with their fingers or rolling it into small balls. We are told that Hawaiians used to eat as much as ten pounds a day. This amount of starch contributed greatly to the obesity of some Hawaiians, which was greatly admired by them. Westerners may find that *poi* tastes a good deal like library paste. At a luau the leaves of the *taro* are also eaten.

Charles Heiser, in *Seed to Civilization,* calls the coconut (*Cocos nucifera*) the world's most useful tree. Every part of it is used. The coconut is not really a nut. It is a fruit— a drupe like plums, cherries and peaches. Coconut trees bear from 50 to 100 fruits a year. After they are harvested they are cut in half, the meat is gouged out and left to dry in the sun to make *copra.* The oil is then extracted. This is what we use for making margarine and soap. The "presscake" that is left after the oil is pressed out contains as much as

124

23 percent protein. And it is one of the most complete proteins, nutritionally speaking. That is, like soybeans, the coconut protein comes nearest to protein from animal sources in its nourishing qualities.

The daily diet of the Pukapukans contains about 1,800 calories, including 70 grams of fat, mostly from coconut oil, plus about one tablespoon of sugar and almost no salt.

In Rarotonga there are plenty of shops selling European food, although the people depend on their traditional food for much of their sustenance. They eat about 2,100 calories daily, including about 63 grams of fat and about four tablespoons of sugar. In New Zealand, where the original Maori people are now successfully integrating with the British inhabitants of the islands, the average daily intake of food contains 2,560 calories, 125 grams of fat, about eight tablespoons of sugar and almost four times the amount of salt the Pukapukans eat.

In a well-designed chart Dr. Prior shows what these various diets are doing to the Polynesian people. Among the Pukapukans, almost 7 percent of the men and 21 percent of the women are obese, though almost nobody is grossly obese. Among the Rarotongans, 8 percent of the men and 22 percent of the women are obese. Among the New Zealand Maori, 18.6 percent of the men and 21.8 percent of the women are obese.

The levels of blood cholesterol show a similar rise as you turn from the primitive people to those raised partly on Western food, then to those who are almost completely nourished on Western food. The levels go steadily up.

The incidence of gout is almost non-existent among both of the former groups. It claims 13.3 percent of all Maori men and 2.5 percent of all Maori women living in New Zealand. Diabetes incidence among Pukapukans is 2 percent for men, 4.4 percent for women, 6.2 percent for

Rarotonga men and 9.5 for their women. Among the Maori in New Zealand 11.9 percent of all men have diabetes and 9.3 percent of all women.

High blood pressure figures show that the Rarotonga people have higher average levels than the New Zealand Maoris, while the Pukapukans have "normal" pressure. Heart disease figures follow the earlier pattern, with the figures for New Zealand Maori women almost eight times those of Pukapukan women.

In Rarotonga the diet consists of canned meat, usually corned beef, canned fish, *taro* and rice, bananas, cabbage, onions, tomatoes, coconut sauce. There is also butter, fresh meat and fish for those rich enough to buy them. Bread is available in bakeries. In Rarotonga the women do none of the gardening, so they are mostly sedentary. Their high-starch diet results in obesity.

In Pukapuka, the appestat seems to be set lower, says Prior. There is also much harder physical work for both men and women. Salaried men's wives, who are mostly sedentary, are significantly heavier than the women who work hard getting and preparing food.

Dr. Prior's group is continuing studies of these people. They have come to no firm conclusions yet, but the evidence seems to lend support to the idea that "advanced nations must reassess very critically our use of many things which constitute our environment and quite clearly our habits of work and diet." The quantity of our food, and also the quality, must be studied, says Prior, especially our use of salt and sugar.

Dr. Price in the 1930's found the native Maori in New Zealand using large quantities of food from the sea, along with sea birds which they captured just before they left the nests when the flesh was tender and very fat from the gorging provided by the parent birds. Large quantities of land birds were also available. Because of the temperate climate and the fertile soil, there was an abundance of wild fruit and vegetables.

Before the white man introduced his cheap, convenient diet, the Maori selected certain shellfish because of unique nutritive attributes which they possessed. While the Prices were in New Zealand they visited a school where, as might be expected, they found almost no tooth decay. Dr. Price asked the teacher what the children ate for lunch since they could not go home to eat. When the school was dismissed at noon, the children rushed to the nearby beach. While one group built a fire, another group dove into the water and brought up lobsters which they cooked and ate.

When the Maori came to New Zealand they brought with them plants which had flourished in their homeland. Enough breadfruit and sweet potato had to be grown to last them the year round, so they stored them in underground cellars much like our "root cellars." The root of the bracken fern was the staple starchy food until "Irish" potatoes and wheat flour were introduced by European settlers. The fern roots were beaten to remove the hard outer coats, then cooked over coals.

Here are some of the vegetable foods the Maori ate during their early days in New Zealand:

four kinds of fern root	*Pteris aquilina esculenta*
cabbage tree	*Cordyline australis*
bulrushes	*Typha augustifolia*
horse-shoe fern	*Marattia fraxinea*
tree fern	*Cyathea medullaris*
bush fern	*Polystichum Richardii*
wild cress	*Nasturtium palestre*
sow-thistle	*Sonchus oleraceus*

The top of the trunk of the palm tree, which is eaten raw, was seldom available, since, once the top is removed, the tree dies. But when a tree was blown over or otherwise destroyed, the Maori made a salad of the tasty tender top of the palm. It is now referred to as the million-dollar salad.

The *karaka* (*Cornycarpus laevigata*) has a prolific crop of berries somewhat like plums. The berries are valued for the sake of their seeds which are cracked and eaten. They contain the same prussic acid elements which make apricot pits and some other seed kernels poisonous when raw. So the Maori cooked them in a large earth oven for 24 hours to drive out the poisonous acid. *Hinau berries* (*Elaeocarpus dentatus*) were pounded to separate the pulp from the hard seeds. The pulp was made into cakes and cooked in the earth oven. *Tawa* berries (*Beilschmiedia tawa*) were cooked over the coals like popcorn. They could then be stored.

New Zealand had no animals that could be hunted except for two kinds of bats and the rats which came along in the Maori canoes. The rats which immediately took to the woods became a valuable game food, which could be caught in any of a number of ingenious traps. In berry-eating time they were a special treat, for they had gorged themselves on berries and were fat.

Fish were abundant. Europeans introduced pigs, cattle and sheep. Of the vegetables brought by Europeans, the Maori liked only pumpkins, squash, potatoes and corn. Peas and beans, carrots, parsnips and onions did not appeal to them, so they did not plant them.

Among primitive people in Australia, those living near the sea use fish and shellfish liberally. In the interior they eat wallaby, kangaroo, small animals and rodents. All the edible parts, including the walls of the viscera and the internal organs are eaten, according to Dr. Price. The Great Barrier Reef off the East coast of Australia extends north to within a few leagues of New Guinea. Murray Island is near the north end of this barrier. The fish in the water at times formed such a dense mass that they could be scooped into boats directly from the sea. Fishermen wading in the surf and throwing their spears into schools of fish usually impaled one or several. Dr. Price found that the incidence of tooth decay on this island was less than one percent of all teeth examined.

Edward Moffat Weyer in *Primitive Peoples Today* describes the austere life of the Arunta, a wandering tribe of the Australian desert, who more closely resemble Neanderthal man than any other human beings today. A perfect example of Stone Age man, they are nomads who have no agriculture, no cooking utensils of any kind, no metals, no bows or arrows. They hunt with boomerangs. In seasonal shifts from warmth to cold, they experience the difference between subsistence and famine. They are never far away from starvation.

The women use digging sticks to get at edible roots or to find burrowing lizards. They dig up the nests of the honey ant and bite off the nectar-filled abdomen. The men hunt kangaroos or emus with spears or boomerangs. The Arunta have no way to carry or store water in this desert country. They must find a waterhole and drink there. Then they poison the water, so that, when the emu comes to drink, he will die and they will have food. The Arunta also eat sweet gum from the *mulga* tree. They have a narcotic, a plant whose leaves they chew for a "high." Dr. Weyer says their appetite for fat is never satisfied. When they kill a kangaroo they pull out the intestines first, looking for bits of fat which they eat immediately. The intestines are then cooked by rolling them in hot ashes.

In the New Hebrides, northeast of Australia, yams—20 varieties of them—form the basis of the diet, along with breadfruit. Yams are not the vegetable our markets sometimes label as yams. Ours are a kind of sweet potato. The South Pacific yam is from a different family, *Dioscorea*. They are eaten for their tuberous roots which may be very large, the flesh colored white, red, gray or dappled. Yams are harvested some five months after being planted. Every tuber planted will, by this time, have increased to six tubers. They contain a good deal of starch and up to 3 percent protein, with considerable potassium and other minerals.

Nineteen varieties of breadfruit are grown on these islands. One kind or another is ripe at almost any time. The islanders did not plant them. They planted themselves. Breadfruit (*Artocarpus altilis*) is a member of the mulberry family. The handsome tree grows 40 to 60 feet tall. The fruit may attain as much as 10 pounds in weight and one foot in diameter. Breadfruit is only about 1½ percent protein, the rest is carbohydrate, with some B vitamins and minerals. Seedless breadfruit is generally prepared by boiling and baking.

Sugar cane is planted with the yams, three kinds of cane. Eleven kinds of bananas are also found among the yam plants. The cabbage bush has red and purple veined three-fingered leaves which are used to wrap foods for cooking. Aside from these vegetarian foods, the New Hebrideans eat crayfish, squid, lobsters, turtles and turtle eggs. They catch fish at night, using flaming torches to scare them into the nets.

The fascination the breadfruit tree had for the British explorers accounts for Captain Bligh's famous trip on the Bounty. He captained a ship sent to bring breadfruit trees back to England where they would be studied as possible food for the West Indian slaves. The Bounty never made it back to England, but Captain Bligh did. He made other trips to the South Pacific where another tree was named for him

—the *Blighia sapida,* or *akee.* The fruit is edible if you pick it at just the right moment. Unripe or overly ripe, it can kill you.

The British were attracted to the idea of a tree which would produce enormous fruit, readymade, apparently growing without any cultivation or effort on the part of the farmers. They simply had to wait until the enormous fruit dropped from the trees. Breadfruit tastes nothing like bread. It is always eaten cooked, never raw, and tastes, says one American traveller, rather like roast chestnut with a slight raisin flavor.

In the Fiji Islands, a garden might contain yams and *kava, manioc,* sweet potatoes, *kawai* and *bulow,* which are smaller starchy roots, plus bananas and eggplant, tomatoes, papaya, a few bushes which produce spinach-like leaves and a few stalks of corn. Bananas are the staple food of the poor. They are picked long before they are ripe and then boiled. They are almost tasteless. Bananas would be offered to a guest if there were nothing else to offer, though most Fijian families serve them every day.

Other staple foods are chestnuts, *dawa* (similar to plums), Tahitian apples, mandarin oranges, lemons, mangoes, guavas, pineapples, and sugarcane. Many varieties of yams grow wild and can be had for the digging—with a stick. Careful, skillful diggers may be able to find and carry home as much as 150 pounds of yams on one trip.

The Fiji Islanders eat chickens, but eggs are considered not fit to eat. In olden times the island had many snakes which were an excellent source of protein food. When European settlers landed, they were horrified at all the snakes. They imported mongooses which rapidly ate all the snakes, then started on the birds' eggs. Now the wild pigeons, which used to be a nutritious item of diet, have also disappeared.

Fijians are fond of a fat grub which is allowed to drink

131

its fill of sweetened coconut milk as preparation for being eaten. It is found in pieces of rotten firewood. Fish and eels, snails and pràwns are eagerly sought.

Puddings may be made of boiled *taro* or breadfruit and coconut. *Taro,* boiled and pounded to a rubbery mass and made into little balls, is dipped in a sweetened liquid squeezed from grated coconut. The coconut has been seared with a hot stone to give it flavor. The little balls are then rolled in coconut gratings and eaten.

A baked pudding made of a sweetened coconut preparation is wrapped in banana leaves and baked in an oven. *Taro* pudding may be made of grated *taro,* pressed into balls, tied in banana leaves, then baked for four or five days. *Manioc,* grated and boiled with grated bananas, makes a kind of porridge served with coconut cream. *Manioc,* pounded with grated coconut and allowed to ferment before baking, makes a kind of "bread" which keeps for many days.

Dr. Price found great immunity to tooth decay among the Fijians when he visited them. They also had well formed faces and dental arches. He could find almost no tooth decay among those who were still eating the native plants and animals. Among those eating "modern" foods the decay ranged as high as 30 percent of all teeth. The cause, according to Price, is the white flour, sugar, sweetened foods, canned foods and rice, brought to the islands by Europeans.

In old-time Samoa, plenty of fish and shellfish were always available for eating, as well as snakes, lizards and land crabs. The Samoans raised pigs and chickens. They had coconut, breadfruit, and banana trees. They planted *taro* and yams, and the little-esteemed sweet potato, as well as paper mulberries and *Pandanus utilis* whose fibers are used for making baskets and mats. Arrowroot, *kava* and sugar cane were other crops. Women weeded and harvested the crops. Men cleared the land and planted.

The Samoan oven was a shallow pit. Round stones were heated, ashes raked away and food placed on the stones, covered with leaves and allowed to bake for an hour or so. The primitive Samoans boiled water by dropping heated stones into wooden pots full of water, then cooked food in the water. They ate coconut raw, but breadfruit, yams, *taro* and bananas were always thoroughly cooked.

Primitive inhabitants of Tasmania were nomads. Each tribe followed animal migrations, says Murdock in *Our Primitive Contemporaries,* the women carrying the household utensils and the children who were too young to walk. They stayed in frail shelters, nothing much more than windbreaks which they abandoned when they moved on in a day or two. They hunted possums, kangaroos, wallabies, bandicoots and wombats. They sought out oysters, crabs and other shellfish, but, for some reason, considered fish as tabu and did not eat it. Wild plants, roots, seeds, berries, fruits, mushrooms and birds' eggs, along with snakes, lizards, ants and grubs made up the rest of their diet.

In *The Road My Body Goes,* Clifford Gessler describes the feast which was held on his first night on the island of Tepuka in Tahiti: pickled raw fish dipped in sweet-salty coconut sauce, freshwater shrimp in fermented coconut, mountain bananas, sweet potatoes, baked breadfruit, two kinds of Tahitian *poi* (which differs from Hawaiian *poi*)—all dipped into coconut milk which had been squeezed out of the grated pulp and salted.

There was little breakfast in Tepuka, he says. The people lived from day to day. Food was scarce until the men came back from fishing. But everyday food might include raw clams, coconut, the tips of the pandanus tree, cooked fish, shellfish, octopus or pounded shark.

Dr. Price says that in some parts of the South Pacific he found much dietetic value placed on fish eggs, especially for growing children. The *angelote* or angel fish (a kind of shark) bears live offspring ready to swim and forage for food from the moment of birth. The eggs of the female were used for food. A pair of glands from the male were especially valued as food for men.

The responsibility of modern processed foods for contributing to tooth decay is amply illustrated in Dr. Price's stories of South Pacific islands where trading ships called for dried *copra* when its price was high for several months. They paid for the *copra* with white flour and sugar. When the price of *copra* went down, the ships stopped calling at these ports and the rampant tooth decay induced by the refined goodies stopped almost at once. Dr. Price examined many of these teeth on such islands and found that the entire decay process stopped when the people went back to their ancestral foods.

Christmas Dinner
on Pitcairn Island

Pitcairn Island is a tiny speck in the South Pacific
Ocean, some one hundred miles from the nearest island.
Less than one mile wide and two miles long, it is a volcanic
island with rich, fertile soil and plentiful rainfall. Its steep
cliffs and precipices rise 1,100 feet above sea level. It is the
home of one of the most interesting and isolated groups of
humanity alive in the world today—the descendants of the
mutineers of the Bounty, early Englishmen whose 18th
century mutiny has been immortalized in books and movies.

Recently Ian M. Ball, an Australian newspaperman
turned New Yorker, visited Pitcairn Island because of his
interest in the Bounty mutiny. He wrote a book, *Pitcairn:
Children of Mutiny,* the first part of which tells the story of
the mutiny. His extensive research on the story convinced
him that Captain Bligh, whom we have always been told
was the villain of the piece, was really a fine captain and the
true villain was Fletcher Christian, leader of the mutineers.

The second part of the book describes the visit of Ball
and his family to the island. Because of its isolation it provides a perfect laboratory for study of a group of people
almost uninfluenced by "civilization." The 85 Pitcairners
who now live on the island are almost all descended from

135

the mutineers who landed from the Bounty 200 years ago. They brought with them Tahitian women and started families. Their descendants have intermarried, which, according to our knowledge of genetics, should have produced dreadful ills in the way of inherited diseases and disorders, both mental and physical.

Instead, Ball tells us he found on the island a group of people "both stoic and good." Deeply religious and involved in the communal life of the island, they "shine in their unselfishness and their spirit of cooperation," he says. There are no degenerative conditions that are noticeable and no diseases typical of the island. Once, years ago, when the islanders rescued a group of ship-wrecked sailors with typhus, they suffered an epidemic which killed 12 Pitcairners. But no other communicable disease has afflicted them, aside from tuberculosis which has taken a few victims.

The Pitcairners' health is not absolutely perfect. They have some asthma, some flu and colds and many problems with sprains and infected cuts resulting from the hazards of their sea-going life. A few Pitcairners have a touch of high blood pressure.

Children are born healthy and alert, although their mothers have no doctors or obstetricians. "In summary, then, today's Pitcairners, after seven generations of intense inbreeding, are basically healthy, strong and alert individuals. (They have terrible teeth, granted, but so, too, do peers of the English realm who provided one-half of their ancestors)," says Ball.

In 1876 the Seventh Day Adventist Church of California sent literature to Pitcairn Island which was read by all the islanders. Although they had been firm Church of England devotees, they gradually became interested in the precepts of the Adventists. In 1886 an Adventist minister came to Pitcairn; within six weeks he had persuaded most of the Islanders of the benefits of this belief. In 1890 the entire community was baptized into the Adventist church. Ball tells us that, "from that time on, the children of the mutineers grew up with minds directed into only two avenues of thought: survival and Christian rectitude, the stomach and soul." Vegetarianism is a basic precept of the Adventist church, but it is not mandatory for Adventists.

In the current Adventist pastor's home, where strict vegetarianism prevails, the Balls were served glutenberger "steaks" and "cold cuts" from a soybean sausage. With these were rolls, vegetables, three salads including one of grated carrots and coconuts, three fruit juices, cakes and fruit salad for dessert. The pastor explained to Ball that Adventist diet rules are principles, not laws.

"We don't regard meat-eating as a sin," he said, "particularly in a place like this where food supplies are short. It becomes a personal matter. You eat first the best things, then the next best and so on . . ."

In the tiny Co-op store on the island, which is open only two hours a week, there are some imported canned foods on the shelves: bully beef, ox tongue, a sausage with vegetables. Although Pitcairners are said to come close to the Adventist church's ideal of vegetarianism, Ball says that most of them are "ravenous meat-eaters." Other cans on the shelves seemed to be only for status, for surely on an island with rich, deep soil and a subtropical climate no one needs canned tomatoes, canned peas, beans, peaches.

In fact, says Ball, there is more perfect, luscious, nourishing food lying around on the ground and hanging, ripe, on the trees than there is in the store. The children pelt one another with ripe mangoes. Custard apples and ripe bananas, oranges, lemons and limes hang on the trees or lie crushed underfoot. There is such a plentitude of fruit that the Islanders can't use it all.

Fish is, of course, a staple food on the island. And since shellfish are forbidden foods on religious grounds, the islanders catch immensely big crayfish and use only the tail meat as bait for catching the fish they are allowed to eat—rock cod, snapper, gray mullet, kingfish. and other fish with fins and scales.

The Balls were invited to a birthday party. There were 42 different dishes on the table, including goat and chicken meat, warm in their cooking pots, plus bully beef and tongue in the cans in which they arrived at the island. Pickfish is a traditional dish, made by picking into tiny pieces any whitefleshed fish, then frying it with an equal amount of chopped scallions.

There were sardines, white and sweet potatoes, string beans cooked in coconut milk, stewed tomatoes, carrots, bananas, cabbage, baked pumpkin, baked beans, butter, homemade bread and biscuits, tomato, cucumber, cabbage and lettuce salad, all with coconut milk dressing. The celebrated local dish, which the Balls found unappetizing, is called *pillhai*, made by baking mashed green bananas in envelopes of banana leaves.

Desserts were fruit gelatins, pumpkin pies, sliced peaches, cakes, buns, cookies. Beverages were fruit juices: peach, pineapple and lemonade. The Balls' hostess on the island, Millie Christian, has a favorite dish which sounds unbelievable: a bowl of homegrown cantaloupe and avocado. She chops them and mixes them with hot baked beans! She drinks only water, "God's water from the well," she says.

For Christmas Dinner on Pitcairn Island the Balls were guests of Tom and Betty Christian. The goodies filled every inch of space on the oilcloth tablecloth. There was goat-meat stew, chicken baked with tomatoes, corned beef, fried goat liver, baked pumpkin, sweet corn, beets, roast potatoes, sweet potatoes, cold canned peas, imported butter, homemade bread, cabbage, tomato and cucumber salad with coconut milk dressing, homemade apricot juice, sour-orange-lemonade and juice from wild strawberries. Dessert was a plum pudding with custard sauce, and wild strawberries with a dish of ice cream made from powdered milk. No hot drinks are served in this abstemious household, except Ovaltine or Milo—both considered "non-stimulating."

Ball recounts one incident when he was walking with a Pitcairn neighbor and they stopped to rest. The islander casually ate four sun-warm pineapples, then sliced up and ate a small watermelon—all this as a snack between breakfast and dinner!

Ball tells us that a Texas physician, Dr. David Gibson, arrived at Pitcairn a month after the Balls left and reported his surprise and gratification at the superb health of the Pitcairners. He examined them, questioned them and then reported, "I am amazed to see 50 and 60 year olds trotting up and down the steep paths of this little island." Men more than 70 years old scramble up rope ladders to the decks of ships.

Ball describes Pitcairn men trundling 200-pound wheelbarrow-loads up the steep cliffs from Bounty Bay with no sign of fatigue. The physical work involved in launching the longboat through the heavy surf every time a ship arrives sounds like something out of the days of galley slaves and pyramid building. All incoming and outgoing freight, too, must be hauled up and down the cliff by ropes or carried through the thick mud of the steep path. No one hesitates for a moment to attack such jobs. In their spare time, and for celebrations, there are lively cricket games played in the subtropical heat. The game which the Balls witnessed was played all afternoon of a day when the islanders got up at 3 A.M. to launch their boats through raging surf to meet a visiting banana boat!

One of the main reasons for the prodigious good health of the islanders must be the vast amount of hard physical labor they put in every day except the Seventh Day which is the Sabbath. We are told that Millie Christian, the Ball's hostess, had, by 11 A.M. served a breakfast of eggs and pineapples to her guests, baked eight loaves of bread in an outdoor, wood-fired oven, finished a pandanus-leaf basket, dyed more pandanus leaves for more baskets, cleaned her house, washed the dishes and prepared another breakfast for her husband—the lunch-breakfast—which consisted of chicken soup with rice and noodles; French fries, pineapples and homemade bread. After doing these dishes, she planned to do the week's laundry by hand!

The men are forever working in their gardens. Gathering and splitting firewood for cook stoves is another hard job which is a daily chore.

So in spite of what was at first assumed to be disastrous interbreeding, in spite of no doctors, no hospitals or clinics, in spite of almost none of the "blessings" of civilization, the Pitcairners are a healthy population. They eat a lot and they work hard physically.

They have apparently no refined carbohydrate except what is brought in by visiting ships. These occasions are so rare that little white flour and sugar makes its way into Pitcairn meals. The abundant tropical fruit, ripened on the trees, satisfies any sweet tooth.

Most of their food is fresh-caught fish, poultry, garden-fresh vegetables and the wealth of fresh tropical fruit which the island provides free the year round. Their religious convictions in regard to food and good health are undoubtedly a major reason for their abundant well-being, as well as their generous, peace-loving natures.

A Visit to the
Stone-Age Tasaday

"And so we two, visitors where none had visited before, sat in silence, dazed as travellers in a time machine might be dazed upon arriving at their most distant destination. Faces appeared in the upper caves. Brown, dark-eyed faces, framed in long black hair. Some smiling, some wide-eyed. We skyborne creatures of man's most advanced and tormented society, and they, perhaps the last of the world's innocents, watched each other across the full span of cultural evolution. And felt love for each other."

With these words, Kenneth MacLeish, senior assistant editor of the *National Geographic Magazine,* described his first sight of the Tasaday, a group of 25 Stone-Age people who live in a remote corner of the rain forest on Mindanao, one of the Philippine Islands. Anthropologists believe that these timid, friendly people may be the last primitive people left to "discover" in our world.

In the *National Geographic,* August, 1972, Mr. Mac-Leish and his photographer report on the lives these people have lived for perhaps a thousand years, without any knowledge that there are other people in the world, aside from the few neighboring tribes they sometimes hear calling in the forest. We call them "Stone-Age" people because they have never discovered how to make things of metal. They use tools and utensils made of stone. They have nothing made of metal. The rain forest in which they live covers the land with thick shade. Trees 200 feet tall rear through the thick canopy of leaves and vines. The 25 Tasaday live in caves.

Through interpreters from tribes which live some distance away but speak a language like that of the Tasaday, the Americans were able to converse with these gentle people. There are ten men; five of them with wives. The rest of the Tasaday are children. The Tasaday told MacLeish that they had always lived where they live today. "We know of no other place where Tasadays have ever lived. Our ancestor had a very good dream there; he told us never to leave that place. There we would have only small coughing, but if we left we would be sick."

What do such forest people eat, having no weapons to kill game, no tools with which to plant crops, no utensils in which to store food? They eat probably very much what our own ancient ancestors ate when they were "Stone-Age people." Their staple food is the wild yam, plus everything edible that they can find in the many streams in which they search regularly for frogs, tadpoles, crabs, little fish. They also eat berries and flowers, wild bananas and the grubs that live in rotten logs.

Some five years previously a member of another tribe visited them and brought them some traps and knives. Until that time they had never killed animals for food. "Our ancestors were friends of the deer and could touch them," they told the visitors.

Their helpful neighbor taught them to make traps in which they could kill deer, wild pigs, monkeys and mice. He taught them to smoke the meat so that it would keep. But, they say, they do not really need the meat. They have enough to eat without it. He also gave them a *bolos,* a heavy knife commonly used in the Philippines. With this they can get what is now their favorite food—*ubud* and *natok.* These are the pulp of two palm trees. With the knives they slit open the trees and get the pulp. *Ubud* tastes like artichoke hearts, says MacLeish. The Tasaday eat it raw. *Natok* must be pounded, strained and cooked. It is hard work, they say, but *natok* has become their favorite food. They do not cut *ubud* near their caves, for they believe that this might make the weather turn bad.

The Tasaday go out every day gathering food. It takes them only a few hours to get all they need. They catch tadpoles, frogs and crabs in the rushing streams, wrap them in orchid leaves and put them beside hot coals to cook. Their wild yam (*biking*) is not like the sweet potato which is called yam in some parts of the United States. It is a large root which the Tasaday dig from the ground with a sharp digging stick. While they are digging the yam or *biking,* MacLeish tells us, they sing a *biking* song, thanking the plant for giving them this food. The yams are then roasted over hot coals, while the women turn them with bamboo tongs.

MacLeish describes how the Tasaday obtain their *natok.* First they make a sturdy platform of sticks, covered with ferns and leaves which will be the filter. Gutters made of banana leaves will carry off the strained fluid. Men pulverize the pithy core of the palm with bamboo mallets. Then a woman, perhaps with her baby in her arms, tramples the liquid out of it, on top of the leafy filter. A man throws on some water from a ladle made of bark. The fluid runs down into a settling trough. The heavier, starchy part of it settles to the bottom. This is the part the Tasaday eat.

Philosophers have long said that the ideal society is one in which so little time is needed to obtain the necessities of life that one has plenty of leisure. A Tasaday family can

143

gather enough food for six in two hours, within about a five mile area from the caves where they live. The rest of the day is leisure. They play with their children, climb trees and vines and relax.

Anthropologists have theorized that, as soon as any primitive society has enough leisure, they begin to invent things and create a "technology" of sorts. How have the Tasaday avoided this stage of development? MacLeish believes it is because they have everything they want or need except for more women—enough for wives for all the single men. "Everything that they know to be good they find in their forest . . ."

When the visitors went with their Tasaday friends to check the traps they had set in the forest they found them all empty. No one was surprised and no one cared. Apparently they have meat only occasionally. But it is well to remember that they are getting protein from the frogs, tadpoles, crabs and fish which they eat. So their diet seems to be as well-balanced as one could wish.

There are no overweight Tasaday. They are all slim, extremely agile and sure-footed, graceful, affectionate, gentle. Their language, like that of the Eskimo, has no word for war. They know nothing of possessions, greed or envy. They feel no need to gather more food than satisfies their hunger from day to day. They feel that their forest home is infinitely beautiful and they have need for nothing more.

Well aware that the Tasaday are a fragile treasure and that any contact with visitors from the outer world is likely to change them in such ways that they will lose their identity and their culture, the Philippine government is making their rain forest a reserve for them and some neighboring people. The greatest fear is that contact with "civilized" people will bring disease.

The New York Times for October 17, 1971 reports

the fears of Dr. Stanley A. Fred, Chairman of the Anthropology Department of the American Museum of Natural History, that all small primitive tribes face possible extinction soon after they are "discovered" by modern man, either from disease to which they have developed no immunity, from destruction of the natural habitat or absorption of their culture into surrounding cultures.

Most of the remaining Stone-Age people live in the Amazon region of South America and in New Guinea. The Xeta tribe of southern Brazil was discovered in 1956. As "civilization" approached, they were persuaded to work on farms. The few who survived influenza, measles and smallpox were absorbed into the nearby society. They now wear this group's clothing and eat their kind of food.

Other endangered tribes are the Akuriyo, persuaded by missionaries to live in villages, now dying of disease. The Parakans and the Asurini, who were "discovered" during the building of the Trans-Amazon Highway, are also threatened. "I can't think of a single tribe that hasn't been significantly decimated by disease after their initial contact with the outside world," said the curator of South American ethnology at the Museum of Natural History.

Manda, the Philippine official who guided the MacLeish party to the Tasadays' home, pointed out, "Maybe we ought to look back to primitive peoples to find out where the world went wrong. There seems to be a growing sense that it has gone wrong. Maybe we can learn from the Tasadays."

After an affectionate embrace and farewell to their Tasaday hosts, MacLeish said to his photographer, "Our friends have given me a new measure for man. If our ancient ancestors were like the Tasadays, we come of far better stock than I had thought."

Milk Has Nourished Mankind through All the Ages

Once in a while, these days, you encounter someone who hates milk, hates it with such a passion that he has fortified himself with much research, he tells you, proving that milk is food only for babies and that anyone over the age of two has no business drinking milk. If God had meant us to drink milk, he may say, it would grow on a tree or a bush. Any animal's milk is food for that animal's offspring only, and man is doing himself grave harm by drinking it.

Possibly many people down through the ages have felt this way about milk. Certainly there have been many cultures where milk other than human mother's milk was never used. But mostly this was because there was, in such cultures, no way to raise or feed milch animals. Eskimos and other dwellers in the Far North live in a land almost devoid of green fodder. Reindeer, who eat mosses and lichens, have been domesticated as a source of milk in some northern countries.

In any case, we know that milk-drinking goes very far back in human history. Many nations have survived in a state of excellent health drinking milk, sometimes along with an excellent diet, sometimes using milk as almost their only food.

We know from archeological records, that at least 5,000 years ago human beings were drinking milk. The early Greeks used goat and sheep milk. Pliny, the Roman naturalist, thought camel milk was the sweetest. The elk was domesticated and milked in some parts of the world. Yaks and asses, buffalo and camels have given milk to many groups of people in past ages.

Since there was no way to refrigerate milk in early days, butter, sour milk and cheese were probably discovered rather soon after human beings domesticated animals. In early Egyptian tombs a fatty substance found in jars is believed to have been butter. In classical Greece and Rome, butter was considered food for barbarians only, while Greek and Roman gourmets used olive oil as their chief source of fat.

But the Romans also used soured milk, *oxygala,* much like our yogurt, which had a fairly solid consistency. *Melcaby,* another form of soured milk, was made by pouring fresh milk into jars which contained boiling vinegar, then keeping it overnight in a warm place. Their gourmet chefs prepared it with salt, pepper, oil and coriander.

From Neolithic times, when people settled into communities and began to plant and harvest crops, they have made cheese. Egyptians made it, so did the early Greeks and Cretans. Homer talked of a pottage made of barley meal, honey, wine and grated goat milk cheese. The Romans smoked cheeses and imported foreign varieties. They used cheese in bread and cakes. The Greek peasant in classical times had a basic diet of barley pastes and gruel, barley bread, olives, figs and goat milk cheese, washed down with goat milk. Different kinds of cheeses and curds were eaten in ancient Assyria and Babylon. They were served in a variety of shapes, in molds which have been discovered by archeologists.

The dowry of an early Persian princess included 100

milch camels and 100 camels "for burdens." One early Persian king was said to have 1,000 animals which gave milk—goats, sheep, camels, but no cows. These early people seldom drank the milk fresh and sweet. They preferred buttermilk, with the cream skimmed off. Or they might eat the yogurt (the curd) as it was, or beaten with fresh spring water as a foamy drink somewhat like an ice cream soda without the carbonation.

The solid part of milk—the yogurt—was used in many ancient recipes. Mixed with onion, black pepper and herbs, it was a sauce for *shish-kebab.* Adding minced cucumbers and raisins to yogurt, the ancients made a creamy cold soup. Honey or fruit marmalade with yogurt was dessert. Or the soured milk might be served as a salad dressing over crisp cucumbers and radishes, both well-known and widely used vegetables. All these recipes are just as tasty today, using modern yogurt as we make it in our kitchens.

The earliest mention of buttermilk in India occurs in a Sanskrit manuscript, "Tales of Ten Princes." In one story a prince sought a bride by asking all the girls in the neighborhood to cook him a meal, using rice from the bag he had with him. The young lady who won his heart served him buttermilk along with a soup and flavored the rice by dusting it with cinnamon. Yogurt, an ancient food in India, is still eaten in quantities in that country.

Galen, the early Greek physician, treated some illnesses with milk, insisting that when asses' milk was used, the animal must be brought into the sickroom. Considering the dangers of contamination, this seems an excellent though not very practical idea. Later physicians thought that human babies should nurse directly from the milch animal to prevent contamination.

Then there were those who were convinced that the milk a young creature drank would greatly influence the way he turned out. There were apocryphal stories of mother dogs raising pigs which behaved exactly like dogs when they were grown. Might not a child raised on cow's milk turn into something like a cow later on? Of course, there was no way at that time to analyze milk or to discover its nutritive value. In those early days a child whose mother died or could not nurse it died unless a wet nurse or some form of animal milk was available.

As early people congregated in villages and cities, the problems of providing milk to the growing population were immense. Molly Harrison says in *The Kitchen in History* that there was no control over the sale of milk in England, even as late as the 18th century. Brought in from the country in open pails, it was often fresh, just as often sour. Milkmaids carried open cans of milk on their heads, going from door to door while slops and rubbish rained down from upstairs windows. Cows kept in town were housed under appalling sanitary conditions.

Louis Pasteur, who first told the world about bacteria and their important role in food as well as in illness, discovered that, if you heat milk to a low temperature which will destroy most of the bacteria, the milk will keep much longer than raw milk. This is why most of the milk we buy today is pasteurized.

Canned milk was first produced in 1835 and Gail Borden (that famous name in the dairy world) improved on the method by patenting in 1856 what he called condensed milk which had been sweetened. This convenient food became popular with soldiers in the American Civil War. Until scientists realized what was involved in sterilization, sugar was added because it helped to prevent the growth of some bacteria.

The early condensed milk—perfectly safe from contamination—was a much better food than any milk which was then available to most people who did not have their own cows. Cheaper brands of condensed milk were made of skimmed milk, so they contained no vitamin A or D. Children fed exclusively on such milks were bound to suffer deficiencies in these two essentials. Probably this was one reason for an increase in rickets—the vitamin D deficiency disease—in poor communities.

"For the young, milk is an almost perfect food. It is also the most complete single food," writes Dr. S. K. Kon in his book, *Milk and Milk Products in Human Nutrition.* "So, since the dawn of civilization man has used for food the milk of large domesticated animals, the cow, the buffalo, the camel, the mare, the ass, the sheep, the goat, the yak and the llama. All these animals are herbivores and, except for the mare and the ass, ruminants, and it is easy to understand why man has used them and not others."

Animals which live almost entirely on vegetable food are, generally speaking, more docile than carnivores (the meat eaters) and they flourish on foods like grass and hay which human beings cannot eat. Why did no one ever raise pigs for their milk? The mother pig knows how to withhold her milk from anyone but her own offspring. So she could not be milked by human beings.

Cows bred by modern dairymen have a fantastically high milk output compared with that of cows of a century or more ago. It is open to question whether this is beneficial in terms of nutrient content to the human beings who drink the milk. We know that milk from wild animals—reindeer, goats, camels, buffalo—is much "richer"—that is, contains far more non-fatty solids and often more fat than milk from modern dairy cows.

Food eaten by all ruminant animals (those that chew a cud) undergoes intensive fermentation in their various stomachs before it is absorbed. So the nutritional requirements of these animals differ from those of human beings. Bacteria in the first stomach, or rumen, of these animals breaks down the protein in their food and rebuilds it into protein needed by the animal. All vitamins of the B complex are synthesized in this process, so these animals have almost no need for these nutrients in their food.

So whether B vitamins are available in their food or not, the B vitamin content of their milk remains the same. Human mothers, who cannot synthesize all these vitamins, but must get them in food, may feed their babies milk which contains considerably less of the B vitamin complex than cow's milk contains. It depends on the diet of the human mother. If her diet has been deficient in B vitamins, cow or goat milk may be more nourishing for a baby than its own mother's milk.

If cows and other ruminants do not need B vitamins in their food, why should the milk which they manufacture for their own offspring be rich in these vitamins? Because the rumen or first stomach has not developed in calves, so when they are babies they must depend on their mother's milk for protein and B vitamins, as human babies do.

Cows and other ruminants also manufacture their own vitamin C and pass it along in their milk. The human mother also produces milk with vitamin C in it, although she cannot manufacture vitamin C for her own needs. She must get it in food. Most animals (except guinea pigs, apes and a few others) and birds make their own vitamin C. The vitamin C content of all milk is small.

The cow or other dairy animal gets her vitamin D from the action of sunlight on her skin. Animals raised in stalls give milk with much less vitamin D. Dr. Kon believes that no milk can be considered to supply enough vitamin D for a human infant or growing child. This is the reason why dairy milk in our country is usually enriched by ultraviolet radiation to produce vitamin D, usually 400 units per quart. This amount is the recommended daily allowance for everyone.

"Although milk is surpassed by many other foods in its content of any one specific nutrient, it is almost unique as a balanced source of most of man's dietary needs," says Dr. Kon. "Only the whole carcass of an animal, including the bones and the liver, could contribute as much as milk, taken as a single food. Some people, such as the nomadic M'Bororo of West Africa, live for months exclusively on milk."

Milk is a good source of B vitamins and calcium, as well as other vitamins and minerals. Its chief contribution to the diet, however, is its protein content. Dr. Kon points out that this is what makes it such a valuable food for whole nations of people where food supplies are nutritionally inadequate. Vitamins can be made synthetically. Calcium can be added to diets in the form of bone meal or chalk. But protein of high biological value cannot be made in a factory. So milk—especially powdered, skim milk—is precious for feeding children and adults in those parts of the world where hunger stalks the population. Protein is what nutritionists call "the limiting factor" in the diets of those children who are trying to survive and grow on mostly starchy foods. Protein is essential, in sufficient quantity, for good mental and physical health, as well as development and growth.

But milk is "indigestible," some people say. And, of course, there are people who do not like milk and are uncomfortable when they drink it, although most of them have no problem with other dairy products like cheese and yogurt. There is a sound physiological reason why some people cannot, with the best will in the world, digest milk. The explanation is simple, but our scientists were so long in discovering it that many misconceptions arose.

The babies of mammals are born with an inherent

153

ability to drink milk, of course, since this is Nature's only provision for their feeding. An enzyme called *lactase* exists in the baby's digestive tract. Its function is to make milk digestible—any milk. If the baby goes on drinking milk for the rest of his life, as many people do in our part of the world, he does not lose this enzyme. It continues, throughout his life, to make his enjoyment of milk felicitous. In parts of the world where, for various reasons, milch animals are not raised, babies are weaned early in life on other foods. They never taste milk, perhaps, for the rest of their lives. So the enzyme which renders milk digestible disappears from their digestive tracts. If, in later life, they are given milk, they will probably find it "indigestible."

Milk is not used in the Chinese cuisine. Reay Tannahill points out in *Food and History* that, if the Chinese had done as other Eastern countries did and soured the milk into something like yogurt, they would have found that it was not indigestible. The lactose which appears in fresh milk undergoes a change when the milk is made into yogurt or cheese. The person who has no lactose enzymes in his digestive tract can enjoy these foods, even though he cannot drink fresh milk.

If, Tannahill says, the venerable Chinese hygienists believed that milk should not be eaten because it was unhygienic, they would probably have decreed that soured milk was totally inedible and unhealthful. The truth is that the chemistry of soured milk products makes them unusually hygienic, as anyone knows who has used yogurt or the yogurt bacteria to encourage the growth of "friendly" bacteria in the intestine.

If you happen to be one of those people who just can't drink milk, then try yogurt or cheese, either of which contains all the nutrients of milk in a form which will cause no difficulty with digestion. Calcium is an essential mineral, regardless of age. Dairy products are prime sources of this nutrient. Those primitive people who did not use milk got their calcium mostly from eating large amounts of fresh, dark-green leafy vegetables and from chewing bones or boiling them with meat. Today bone meal supplements and other calcium supplements are good sources of this mineral.

Use milk and milk products in meal planning, especially if you are cooking for children or old folks. Its illustrious history as nourishment for man recommends it as the near-perfect food.

Can Man Live on Bread Alone?

"We all live on bread and water," said St. Jerome in the fourth century AD, "a familiar and common practice and we do not t ink it fasting." Ever since human beings discovered how to plant and harvest cereals, people of many countries have depended on bread as the staple food of their diets. Throughout history in most parts of the world, people considered themselves lucky if they could get enough bread to live on, with almost nothing else in the way of food. For famine and starvation have stalked the planet's human inhabitants through all of recorded and pre-recorded history.

In his book *Hunger and History,* E. Parmalee Prentice describes the place of bread in European diet since early times. Bread made of wheat rather than other cereals has always been prized as the best kind of bread. But wheat has greater requirements in regard to soil and fertilizer. So rye was used for bread throughout most of Europe. And as people needed to supplement their flour, they made bread from barley, millet, oats, buckwheat, rice, vetch, beans, peas, lupines, lentils and the bark of trees. In some communities chestnuts provided the staple food and bread as such was a holiday treat.

During famines apparently, tree bark was used as one

ingredient in bread, to eke out a failing supply of flour. In Sweden, as late as 1799, bread was made of the inner part of the fir tree and dried sorrel with no cereal flour whatsoever. It seems unlikely that such a "bread" would resemble in any way our notion of bread. But famine makes strange recipes. It is not surprising that when drought, rainy seasons, blight or insects destroyed grain harvests (and this happened with dismal regularity) many supplementary foods were added to bread as substitutes for unavailable cereal flour.

Before cereals were domesticated acorns were the staple food in some areas of the world. Although many animals, including pigs, love the taste of acorns and will thrive if fed on them exclusively, human beings find these nuts of the oak tree singularly bitter and sour. Many recipes for getting rid of the bitter taste are available in old books. It was an involved, time-consuming process, but acorns were plentiful and free, so all the work seemed worth-while.

Giovanni Battista Segni in a book published in Bologna, Italy in 1602, presents some ways to make bread go farther with differing suggestions for the rich and the poor since, presumably, they would have different ingredients at hand.

Use horse beans, he says (*vicia faba*—now more commonly called broad beans). Use chickpeas, white beans, lentils, millet, vetch, chestnuts, pumpkins, apples, turnips. Add any or all of these to the available flour to make your bread.

He also recommends *polenta,* the Italian dish like our cornmeal mush. For poor people in times of famine he recommends a kind of grass which can be dried in the oven, also acorns, chestnuts, vetch, lupines, Jerusalem artichokes, roots of cabbage, and the dried and pulverized twigs from chestnut and oak trees. He also suggests they might add figs, raisins, pears and a number of herbs to make the whole thing taste better.

It strikes us as strange that people who are supposedly starving are assumed to have on hand such nourishing food as pumpkins, raisins, artichokes, figs and chestnuts, but apparently bread was the backbone of everyone's diet. If one did not have enough bread, he thought he was starving no matter how many vegetables, fruits and wild nuts were available.

Through the ages it appears that bakers and millers have been suspected of all kinds of malfeasance in regard to the manufacture of their products. In 1602 Signor Segni reported that "Some of the bakers who have little conscience (and we have found many such) put in lime or ground earth or chalk." These seem harmless enough additives compared with the chemicals found in some modern foods. But the 17th century bakers also dumped tares (vetch seeds) and dross (rubbish!) into their dough to make it heavier, then represented it as all wheaten bread. Segni claimed that badly risen bread "to deceive us on the weight" had made thousands of people die.

For many centuries French bread has been regarded as the best bread in Europe. But bread in France before the 19th century was quite different from Parisian bread today. Wheaten bread was an expensive luxury. Poor people ate rye bread or bread made from some of the mixtures mentioned above. Even so, bread was the staple food of everyone in France, rich and poor alike. During the famine of 1709 Voltaire mentioned that some rich families were reduced to eating oaten bread, "Madame de Maintenon setting the example."

The size of a loaf of bread was such that one loaf made a meal for even a very hungry man. During the 18th century a loaf of the best Parisian bread weighed 12 ounces. In one part of France loaves of bread weighed 20 to 30 pounds each. They would keep for a month in winter. Goodness knows how anyone managed to hack off a slice of such bread. In another region, it was customary to bake only twice a year. Boys who went to boarding school took a six-month's supply with them. It was so hard it had to be broken with a hammer and soaked before it could be eaten.

When it was fresh, old-time European bread was soft, but as it grew older it became rock-hard. At mealtime in earlier days it was customary to use a slice of hard bread as a "plate" on which softer foods were placed. Thus the gravy or the sauce, the meat juices or any other "sops" were absorbed by the bread and then eaten. The slice of bread was called a *tranchoir,* from which we get the word trencherman —someone who can clean up everything on his plate and then eat the plate!

It is not surprising to discover that in earlier times it was assumed that human beings could live healthfully on bread alone. And, if the bread were whole-grain and eaten in quantity, it would supply plenty of protein, B vitamins and minerals. It is surprising, however, that no one seemed to realize the great importance of other fairly common foods to supplement the bread.

Today we know that bread contains no vitamin A or vitamin C. In northern countries where populations must have been decimated by scurvy each winter, from lack of vitamin C, how did it happen that no one discovered for thousands of years that fruits and fresh vegetables are essential to good health, because of their vitamin C content?

How does it happen that pumpkins and squash—rich in vitamin A—were considered as possible ingredients of bread only under famine conditions? When peas, lentils and beans were used as ingredients, why was the bread considered inferior? Today we know that the protein of these legumes would complement the protein of the cereal flour, to make a

160

high protein bread of good biological value—much more nourishing than plain wheat or rye bread.

We also know that the dark brown, black or gray bread of the peasants, which was "coarse" and not considered worthy of a rich man's table, was also the most nourishing because it was whole-grain. And why was it deemed necessary to make such foods as peas, beans and lentils into bread? Why weren't they just eaten as gruel or mush? Oats, for example, do not make good bread unless it is raised with baking powder which was unknown in those days, or unless it is mixed with plenty of wheat flour in a yeast-leavened bread. Why not use these foods as highly nourishing main dishes, rather than going to all the trouble of making these rather incompatible foods into a form of bread?

Probably one reason was convenience. Bread, solid and long-lasting, could be carried in a pocket all day for eating away from home. It could be, and was, used as a plate. It could be stored for long periods. One needed to build a fire for bread-baking only occasionally, rather than stirring up a new fire every day to prepare mush, lentils or gruel. But, most of all, bread seems to have been a symbol, an elemental link with the earth. Its relatively high protein content made it much more satisfying than low-protein, high-starch foods like squash or fruit.

A large part of mankind, down through several thousand years of history has lived chiefly on bread. He has survived plagues, famines and scurvy so we must believe that good wholegrain bread, in enough quantity, can sustain whole continents of people, provided sources of vitamin A and C are available at least some of the time.

In our era, of course, there is no need to do without all the other valuable foods we have. But bread is still a staple, especially the full-flavored, highly nourishing kind you make at home from first-class, wholesome, unrefined ingredients.

161

The Lowly Potato Has an Honorable History

Dietetic experts these days sometimes treat the humble potato with considerable scorn. They speak disparagingly of "meat and potato diets" as lacking in imagination and essential food elements such as vitamin A. But the potato has a royal ancestry, a glorious history as one of the basic foods of a great number of people who lived in the past.

Potatoes were grown in Chile and the Andes regions of South America long before any Europeans came to this hemisphere. Carleton Beals reports in his book, *Nomads and Empire Builders,* that botanists have classified more than 50 varieties of potatoes grown in one Bolivian valley. On a rainy island off the coast of southern Chile, the Spanish invaders of the 16th century found a group of Indians who planted 100 different kinds of tubers or potatoes as their chief crop. Each variety was entirely different from any potatoes grown on the mainland, where at least 30 kinds of potatoes were grown. Near Cuzco, the seat of the Inca empire, 52 varieties of potatoes were known.

There were white, golden, yellow, black, blue, lead-gray, brown and red potatoes. Beals says that the major varieties are called "races" in Spanish, for they have the characteristics of well-defined stock that cannot be crossed with other varieties. Authorities believe that the beginning of such development and stabilization probably dates from 5,000 years before Christ. So we are talking about a noble tuber which sustained entire nations as their basic staple food for more than 7,000 years.

The Highland people who lived in the Andes had many ways of preserving potatoes through the long, cold winters. In many parts of South America potatoes were, and are still, preserved by a process of freezing and dehydrating. Makers of present-day frozen, dehydrated foods might remind themselves that they have invented nothing new. Primitive South American Indians have been using the same process for many thousands of years.

The potatoes were harvested, then taken to high, open ground and spread out. They were sprayed with water many times and allowed to freeze. Then they were dried. The dried, frozen potatoes were then trampled on grass beds until they were reduced to small black marbles called *chuño,* which means "frozen" in the Aymara Indian language. These "marbles" can be stored and will keep for years without spoiling. In many parts of South America the same process is followed today. The *chuño* are stored and used throughout the winter. They are pulverized for soup, purée, mush, sauces and puddings.

Potatoes to be eaten fresh were stored in llama-wool bags. Seed potatoes were stored in stone bins with straw linings and treated with an herb which prevented rot and sprouting, a technique which modern agronomists should investigate. In our sophisticated age, modern agribusiness uses poisons to inhibit sprouting.

The early South Americans also used potatoes for medical purposes. Since a fresh, raw potato contains considerable amounts of vitamin C, it is understandable that it might have performed what appeared to be miracles of healing.

The Indians used potato poultices on broken bones and rubbed slices of raw potato on their temples to cure headaches. They rubbed healing wounds with *chuño* flour mixed with powdered brick and vinegar, to prevent scars. Potatoes were ground with willow ash and olive oil to prevent rabies.

Potatoes retain heat well, so they were used for poultices to alleviate gout, cure rash, pimples, erysipelas and other skin disorders. Legend has it that you could carry three potatoes (presumably *chuño* rather than fresh) in your pocket to prevent rheumatism. And if you ate slices of raw potato with meals you would never have indigestion.

The South American Indians had names for their potatoes which gave vivid pictures of each variety's attributes. There was "Knife-Breaker," a potato so hard it couldn't be cut until it was cooked. And "Gray-Feather" which must have been shaped and tinted like that. There were "Bird-Egg," "Red Mother," "Human-Head." One with reddish flesh was called plaintively "Weeps Blood for the Incas."

In their book, *Foods America Gave the World,* Verrill and Barrett report that "The display of potatoes in a Peruvian market is simply bewildering. There are tubers with white, yellow, pink, gray and lavender 'meat,' with skins white, pink, red, yellow, brown, green, purple, orange, black and spotted and streaked with various hues; potatoes of every conceivable size and shape, some as smooth and shiny as a tomato, others as rough and warty as a toad."

Some of the potato plants grow three or four feet in height, others sprawl on the ground. They have flowers of rainbow shades. And, most important of all, there are varieties adapted to every kind of soil and climate. They will grow in sunny, fertile valleys, in the damp tropical lowlands or the bleak mountain plateaus.

Spanish explorers took potatoes back to Spain, then brought them back to Florida when they colonized there. Sir

Francis Drake and Sir Walter Raleigh brought potatoes to the British Isles from Florida. From Spain cultivation of potatoes spread slowly to Italy, the Low Countries, Austria, Germany, Switzerland and France.

Although potatoes are cheap, tasty, easy to grow, versatile and nourishing as food, Europeans were slow to adopt them as a common food. They looked unappetizing, people thought, and rumors spread that potatoes, which are after all members of the deadly nightshade family, might be the cause of leprosy, fevers or other illness.

An English physician wrote of them in 1650: "Potato-roots are of a temperate quality and of strong nourishing parts; the nutriment which they yield is, though somewhat windy, very substantial, good and restorative, surpassing the nourishment of all other roots or fruits . . . they are very pleasant to the taste and do wonderfully comfort, nourish and strengthen the body."

But only in poverty-stricken Ireland did they rapidly become popular food. So, of course, when British colonists came to the New World, they brought with them seed potatoes for planting "Irish" potatoes, and that is how they came by this name. The word potato, incidentally, is a corruption of *batata,* which is the Indian name for the sweet potato, an entirely different family of foods. The Inca name for the white (or Irish) potato is *papa.*

Before the mid-eighteenth century, potatoes were a common food among the poor in all of Europe, mostly it seems because the poor could not afford to buy spices to flavor their food. Rich people, who smothered everything they ate in spices and herbs, found potatoes tasteless, uninteresting. So, just as the poor were forced to eat whole grain breads while the rich had the "luxury" of white flour, so the poor got all the nutritional benefits of the new vegetable which was too bland for rich gourmet diners.

166

Then, too, we are told that mankind had lived so long on bread, 200 years ago, that there was a tendency to value any new foods by their suitability for use in bread. And sure enough, some enterprising cooks came up with recipes for potato bread which was a dismal failure. Meanwhile the Germans were distilling "spirits" (perhaps vodka?) from potatoes, using the residue as animal food. Potatoes were also used as they are today, for making flour, starch and syrup, according to contemporary writers.

The many varieties of potatoes which were grown in earlier times and even today in South America may well contain greater amounts of vitamin C, the B vitamins and potassium than our present-day potatoes. Today our agronomists develop potatoes, as they do other vegetables and fruits, for ease in harvesting, for resistance to blight and insects, and for endurance in storage. Earlier potatoes, bred with no such qualifications in mind, could have contained far more nutriment.

We do not take seeds from potato plants, as we do with other vegetables. Instead "seed potatoes" are planted. The potato shares its family relationship with a number of poisonous relatives, as well as wholesome vegetables such as eggplant, tomato, green peppers and chili peppers. Tobacco and petunias are also members of the Nightshade family.

Today potatoes are probably our best known and best liked vegetable. They are so versatile that they can accompany almost any dish. The French discovered how to fry them in deep fat and French Fries and potato chips became best sellers in modern times. To get the full nutritive value of potatoes bake or boil them. Most of the nutrients, which are located just under the skin, are lost when potatoes are peeled raw. If you soak them, nutrients leach out. If you plan to mash potatoes or use them in salad, leave the skin on while you cook them, for you can then remove just the

167

skin, leaving intact the nutrients directly beneath it.

Potatoes are chiefly valuable for their vitamin C and vitamin B content, along with a goodly supply of the mineral potassium. Baked or boiled, they contain almost no fat and only about 20 percent carbohydrate. A medium-sized boiled or baked potato has only about 80 to 90 calories, so the calorie-counter's abhorence of potatoes seems unjustified.

Wouldn't cooking and eating be more interesting if we had as many varieties of potatoes to choose from as those ancient, uneducated, "backward" South American Indians had?

Let's Eat the Bugs!

For many years forests in the Northeastern part of the United States have been ravaged by gypsy moth caterpillars. Several kinds of pesticides have been sprayed from the air in some regions, over the protests of conservationists. And the gypsy moth has moved inexorably on to greener forests. In 1973 residents in the Pocono Mountains vacation area urged the state to return to the use of the proscribed DDT, to combat the moths.

In some localities caterpillars were ankle deep on the ground. Summer visitors were nauseated. Squeamish people dared not venture out of their homes.

Our early ancestors and many groups of primitive people alive today regarded insects as very good food, delicacies, you might say. Why shouldn't we? Why should we continue to devastate our land with poisons, year after year, in order to destroy what is surely one of our best sources of protein—in a protein-hungry world! Surely anyone who has ever eaten a snail, an oyster, or a dab of caviar has no excuse for feeling squeamish or queasy over a fine fat grub.

In *Food and Antiquity,* Don and Patricia Brothwell remind us that primitive man acted on the principle that he should eat anything that was edible. He caught and ate every kind of bug, adults and larvae, winged and terrestrial, pests and beneficial ones alike.

In remote regions of Australia, today, many insects are available and eaten during the rainy season, ants and termites the year round. A sweetish excretion of the larvae of *psyllid* insects, which can substitute for sugar, is found on eucalyptus leaves. The honey-ant (*Melophorus inflatus*) gathers honey in her abdomen until it has grown to massive size, then starts back to home base with it. Any industrious gatherer of food can catch the ponderous ant, bite off the abdomen and enjoy a delicious snack.

The *Bugong* moth (*Euxoax infusa*) and the Ghost moth are eaten by primitive Australians. They also eat beetle larvae and many kinds of caterpillars. Like people in other parts of the world, they relish "locusts," a word which refers usually to any member of the grasshopper family with short antennae. The aborigines remove the legs and wings and roast the creatures.

Early cave drawings show bees and grasshoppers being eaten. Aristotle, in classical Greece, spoke of the larvae of the cicada group as tasting best when they were fully grown. The adult females were best when they were full of eggs, he thought. The Brothwells tell us that the grasshoppers which were sold in ancient Greek markets were bought mostly by the poor. But large oak grubs were considered such a gourmet treat that they were domesticated and fattened on flour.

Members of the grasshopper family came in vast hordes to devour the crops of early farmers. Why not capture and eat then? In Leviticus, the Bible gives full permission to eat the bugs, "the locust after his kind, and the bald locust after his kind and the grasshopper after his kind."

Restaurant keepers in China in the days of Marco Polo served silkworms made into pies, which were much like their shrimp pies. Grasshoppers were eaten by poor Chinese peasants, although they were called "brushwood shrimp" as a euphemism, much as a Chinese peasant, sitting down to a meal of fried rat, called it "household deer."

African pygmies collect and eat termites and colonial caterpillars. They have worked out careful methods of harvesting them. They measure the termite hills to see how high up the insects have risen inside and how soon they will swarm. Each family sets up a windscreen, builds a roof of leaves, digs a deep trench at the base, then builds a fire in front of the trench and a hole in front of the fire.

When the termites begin to fly, they fall into the hole from which the women scoop them in baskets. They are eaten raw or roasted. Or they are pounded into a paste and boiled. The oil that rises to the top of the utensil is skimmed off and used for cooking or as a cosmetic.

Indians in Northern Nevada hunted crickets in somewhat the same way. They dug trenches 30 feet long, joined at the ends, facing uphill and covered with stiff grass. Then swinging fans of grass, they drove the crickets toward the trenches. As the insects crawled into the grass for cover, the Indians set fire to the grass—and presto—roast crickets for dinner!

Dr. Price mentioned the many insects which his hosts on many continents used as basic foods. So important are caterpillars to the Bantu people in Africa that, when they migrate from the bush into town, it has been found necessary to ship in caterpillars, cook and package them, and sell them in food stores. They provide protein, as all food of animal origin does, plus B vitamins in abundance, and many minerals. It's safe to say, if the Bantu town-dwellers are faced with eating the refined, processed, carbohydrate-rich foods which are so inexpensive and easily available in markets, the caterpillars may well be the single most nutritious item in their meals.

171

The Aztec Indians in Mexico ate practically anything that lived in lake water, including the larvae of water flies and insect eggs which they skimmed off the surface of the water and ate like caviar. Why not? They also extracted grubs from the fresh leaves of the maguey cactus, which they considered delicacies. Verrill in *Foods America Gave the World,* describes the big, smooth-skinned larvae of certain Sphinx moths or Hawk moths which are dropped by South American Indians into boiling fat. The grubs puff up, turn crackly brown and look like fritters. The flavor and texture are much like that of soft shell crabs.

South American Indian nations depended on grasshoppers for a large part of their food supply, according to Verrill. They dried them, removed legs and wings and pounded them into a mash which was used as cakes or "bread," or put in soups. In the West Indies grubs of a large weevil which inhabits a palm tree were roasted on spits over open fires. They popped open like roasted chestnuts which they resembled in flavor. In Mexico, Verrill bought insect eggs in markets. The egg masses of aquatic insects tasted to him like unsweetened tapioca pudding.

And right here in the USA in the most unexpected places insect eating is indulged in—and for the most unexpected reasons.

E. J. Kahn, Jr., in *The Big Drink, The Story of Coca Cola,* tells us that the curator of Emory University Museum was a star witness in Coca Cola's court cases where aggrieved consumers reported on various insects they had found at the bottom of Coke bottles. Dr. Fattig told many a courtroom that the bugs were quite dead and rendered harmless by the carbon dioxide in the brew. Then, to emphasize his point, "publicly and blandly consumed some ten thousand stone-cold gastronomic oddities, including flies, fleas, grasshoppers, wasps, praying mantises, beetles, caterpillars, earthworms, centipedes and stink bugs. When one plaintiff's lawyer intimated that his client had been undone by a critter that had somehow survived its immersion in Coke, Fattig calmly popped a live black widow into his mouth and chewed it up."

Of course we are told that Emory University receives vast sums in grants from Coca Cola, so Dr. Fattig's self-sacrifice is perhaps not so unexpected after all.

There doesn't seem to be much sense to eating insects if it turns out that they are just fiber and starch. But, not surprisingly, they are made up almost entirely of protein, as we are. Accompanying that protein is a goodly supply of minerals and vitamins. The Brothwells assert that termites, fried lightly and eaten as they are in the Belgian Congo, were found to contain 44 percent fat and 36 percent protein. A serving (about 3½ ounces) contains some 560 calories. They are also rich in phosphates. For comparison, a broiled sirloin steak is 32 percent fat and 23 percent protein, with 387 calories.

Silkworm pupae, which are now being eaten in some parts of the world, have 23 percent protein and 14 percent fat. The dried locusts or grasshoppers which are eaten by many people in remote parts of the world, have 75 percent protein and 20 percent fat. For comparison, a 3½ ounce serving of boiled soybeans (whose protein is not quite as nourishing, biologically speaking, as animal protein) gives you only 11 percent protein and 6 percent fat, with 130 calories.

The locusts provide, in addition, 1.75 milligrams of the B vitamin riboflavin and 7.5 milligrams of niacin, another B vitamin. A serving of fried liver (our best source of riboflavin) gives you 4 milligrams and 16 milligrams of niacin.

To primitive people the calorie content of such fatty food was very important, for they worked hard physically

173

to make a living out of what was, very often, a hostile environment where food was mighty scarce. We are presently approaching a period of worldwide scarcity of food, we are toid by a number of knowledgeable experts. Refer to Georg Borgstrom's *Too Many* or Paul Ehrlich's *Population Bomb,* as starters.

Experts in the Food and Agriculture Organization of the U.N. and in universities all over the world are working feverishly with brewer's yeast, powdered milk, soybeans, fishmeal, leaf protein, petroleum products and dozens of other relatively inexpensive foods and non-foods, trying to concoct some highly-concentrated nutrients which will be acceptable to people who appear to be the ones who will go hungry or starve before the rest of us do—primarily the people in the undeveloped countries. Population in these nations is doubling in the exponential way which guarantees huge numbers of people who seem destined to starve sooner or later.

Everywhere in the world insect pests take a large part of any given harvest. In our country, in spite of the vast amounts of pesticides in which we drench so much of our agricultural land, we still lose precious food to insects. As well as forests and plains.

If African pygmies can devise ingenious ways to capture practically all the termites in a given hill, and Nevada Indians had methods for luring enough crickets to roast and eat for many days, surely the engineers of our modern technological world can contrive ways of capturing the insect pests that devastate so much of the earth.

And surely American food technology, which gave us the Space Bar, the candy bar, the muffin mix and Seven-Up, can invent ways to make this highly nutritious insect windfall palatable to almost anyone anywhere. We can grind it up, flavor it and make a delicatessen meat out of it. Or dry

174

it into powder and make it into bread. It could be liquefied, bottled and sold as an exotic milk, or made into melba toast, crackers or crackerjack.

I am not suggesting that you pick up the nearest woolly bear caterpillar and sample it, or that you handpick all the mites, scales and spiders from your houseplants and pop them into your mouths. Or, God forbid, that you order a pint of ladybugs for the purpose of making canapes.

There may be insects in one form or another which contain substances toxic to man. We need the advice of entomologists as to which bugs are edible and in what amounts. Once we have that, why not call out the Boy Scouts or the recycling group when the next plague of gypsy moth caterpillars shows up, or canker worms, or spruce bud worms or tent caterpillars or saw fly or tussock moth caterpillars, and turn the kids loose on the bugs? It would be hardly more revolting or strenuous than recycling dirty beer bottles.

If the government could set up centers where the bugs could be processed, we could freeze them and send them in. Costs could be shared by the farmers or tree growers whose crops we save or the municipality which is spared the expense of spraying. Of course, the chemical companies would denounce such an effort as anti-American, but who cares?

Let's eat the bugs instead of poisoning them and poisoning the planet in the process!

Chapter
16

Let's Get Acquainted
with the Many Foods
Used by Other Societies

Why did carob flour go so long undiscovered by modern Americans? What about that marvelous sweet fruit, the *mangosteen*, that grows in the Pacific Islands, a fruit for which Queen Victoria offered a prize? Why aren't we eating it today? In books about foods eaten by faraway and ancient people, we read of many kinds of dates. Yet the ones you see in the supermarkets are all the same, taste the same, look the same. Why?

Why doesn't somebody in this country cultivate yams —the tropical kind—so that people in low income brackets might eat them less expensively than baker's bread or doughnuts? Most primitive people have access to 15 or 20 kinds of bananas. Why do we find the same tired, old, yellow speckled ones at the supermarket year after year? And why don't we import more plantains? They are at least as tasty as bananas, yet few Americans have ever tasted them.

Coconuts. Now there's a food which should be used for many things other than trimming the icing on a coconut cake or stuffing a chocolate bar. Coconuts are 3.5 percent protein, considerably more than brown rice. They contain only 9.4 percent starch and 35 percent oil—perfectly natural, unprocessed oil—which makes them fine foods for the low carbohydrate reducing diet. Why can't we devise ways to get them year round, in good condition, with some ingenious recipes for grinding, blending and pureeing them for tasty main dishes? Wouldn't all our diets be better for it?

The Romans of Caesar's time ate gladioli bulbs and the roots of rampion (*Campanula rapunculus*), sometimes 12 inches long and easy to dig. And they ate roots of salsify, madder (*Rubia tinctorum*), elecampane (*Inula helenium*), muscaria (grape hyacinth), Star of Bethlehem (*Ornithaga-lum umbellatum*), Spanish oyster plant, caladium (*Colocasia*), asphodel (*Asphodelus*). Did you ever see any of these listed in the vegetable pages of your seed catalog, let alone on the vegetable counters at the supermarket? Why not? They might turn out to be much more interesting than beets or turnips, asparagus or carrots. Why not plant purslane and make salad of it, as the Georgians do?

The early Romans made a puree of nettles, which must have been a lot like spinach with an egg sauce. Who knows, it might have tasted even better and might turn out to be even richer in folic acid and iron than spinach is. The Romans also ate mallows, hollyhocks and *orach,* defined in our horticulture encyclopedia as French spinach. (And wouldn't *that* surprise our Roman ancestors?)

Most primitive people living near a seacoast ate sea-weed regularly. And of course it is still eaten in Japan. The North American Indians ate lichen when times were hard. What's the nutrient content of lichen, which also nourishes caribou? Does anyone know?

Is there any good reason why we don't eat *Scirpus* bulbs (bulrushes) or water chestnuts, wild chicory, groundsel (*Senecio*)? The Romans used groundsel in salads. This plant family contains hundreds of varieties, among them the beautiful cineraria at our florists' shops.

178

A Roman cook, Columnella, had a basic salad from which he concocted many varieties. The basic ingredients were: savory, rue, mint, coriander, parsley, chives or green onion, lettuce, kale, thyme, catmint and green fleabane. Today most of us think of salad in terms of a lifeless and tasteless leaf of lettuce chopped up and drowned in bottled dressing loaded with chemical additives. How lucky the early Romans were!

In Greece in Pliny's time quinces were considered "golden apples" and much prized. Nowadays it's almost impossible to get a quince unless you are willing to drive out into the country to some old farm where a gnarled, wormy quince tree may still be standing.

The ancient Europeans ate serviceberries (*Ame-lanchier*), raspberries, blackberries, rose hips, elderberries, cornel cherries (*Cornus mas*), rowan berries (the mountain ash), bilberries (*Cavinium caespitosum*), hawthorn berries, bittersweet and dewberries. Today, with all the efficient agricultural methods, ways of preserving fresh food and rapid transportation, I cannot buy any of these berries, fresh, in a supermarket. Even such common delights as raspberries are no longer available, without special trips to the country or the farmers' market. Supermarket strawberries, sometimes available out of season as well as in June, were obviously grown thousands of miles away and have suffered nameless atrocities on their way to the market.

The *medlar* is a fine tree which came from Persia and was cherished in Greece. The fruit, thoroughly ripened, is rumored to be an excellent dessert. It's unlikely that any of us will ever have the opportunity to sample one. The Greeks used to toss apricots into just about everything they cooked, like a fricassee of pork shoulder, for instance. Most fresh apricots we see these days are the hard, knotty, little ones, always picked green and never seeming to ripen. The *Jujube*

179

(*Zizyphus Jujuba*) was the lotus eaten by those far-out languorous people in the Odyssey. It grows in the southern U.S.A. and is still used in Southern Europe as a dessert fruit and in winter as a dry sweetmeat.

The cherimoya (*Annona Cherimola*), says Liberty Bailey in his *Cyclopedia of Horticulture,* is considered by many to be the finest of the subtropical fruits. Many people in different parts of the world are apparently eating it today. But not Americans. The *granadilla,* eaten by early Americans, is the fruit of one kind of passion flower (*Passiflora*) which also goes by the names of Sweet Cup or Bell Apple. Sounds most appetizing to me. Where can I get one?

Breadfruit trees never set seed, so they can be propagated only by sprouts from the roots. The fruit has a consistency somewhere between new baked bread and sweet potatoes. Wouldn't it be a fine addition to our stock of foods —easy to grow, easy to care for and harvest? And it contains as much vitamin C as some varieties of oranges, plus considerable vitamin B.

Mangoes, another almost forgotten fruit in markets in my part of the country, may have been the first tree to be cultivated by human beings. Akbar, the Moghul emperor who reigned in India from 1556 to 1605, had an orchard of 100,000 mango trees. They grow so readily in a forest that it is hard to tell which of the trees you see growing there have escaped from orchards.

Marston Bates, in *Where Winter Never Comes,* proposes guavas as the horticultural challenge of the future. No two varieties are alike. They differ in size, color, flavor and texture—"a mass of material waiting for the hand of the skillful plant breeder," he says. Mostly they grow in dooryards in the tropics. Some of the varieties are so delicious they compare with our finest fruits. Others are hardly worth the trouble of picking.

Their vitamin C content is very high, from 23 to 1,160 milligrams per 100 grams—more vitamin C than other fruits, even acerola or most rose hips. Why are we letting them perish, unmourned, in the dooryards of the tropics?

Bates remarks on the important role fruits play in tropical diets, in spite of the fact that one seldom sees orchards. The only source of the bewildering variety of fruits seen in tropical markets seems to be the dooryards of individual homes.

He believes that one answer to nutritional problems in the tropics is further horticultural work with fruits like guava, to develop superior varieties and to establish them as profitable items of commerce.

On the other hand, in areas where commercial interests have taken over the production of fruit—the pineapple, for example, the ensuing industrialization and plantation agriculture brings dense populations of tropical workers, cut off from their traditional dooryard foraging for fruits. So, for such workers, fruits have become an expensive luxury.

The Polynesians introduced something like 100 different food plants when they arrived in Hawaii. Many of these were propagated by cuttings which had to be carried over long sea voyages in open boats. How many new plants has modern industrialized U.S.A., with its widespread, well-funded agricultural establishment, given to the world?

There is an enormous amount of information available in old books on how to prepare acorns to make them not only edible but tasty as well. Our food technologists, desperately trying to find inexpensive new or old foods (or non-foods) to nourish the future millions or billions of starving people in the underdeveloped world, might keep acorns in mind.

Surely hikers, Boy Scouts, Sierra Club and Audubon Society members could be enlisted to gather them by the ton during their expeditions into the forests. Fewer acorns might mean fewer oak trees congregated in one area which, we are told, would be a healthy thing for the forests, which tend to degenerate when one species dominates the woodland.

The New York Times reported on July 28, 1973 on a tribe of Indians who live in a remote region on the west coast of the Gulf of California, in Mexico's Sonoma Province. These people have as their basic food a grain derived from eelgrass (*Zostera marina*). It grows in seawater and is believed to be very nourishing and low in fats.

The original report in *Science* states that this is the only known instance of grain from the sea being a staple human food, and suggests that, in a world heavily dependent on a limited number of cereals for sustenance, eelgrass sounds like an excellent prospect for development. It can be grown without pesticides or fertilizers which might degrade the environment.

Flour made from eelgrass is bland. The plant grows under water, but as the seeds ripen, the seed heads break loose and float to the surface. By April or late May, says *The Times,* great masses of the material are floating along the shore. The Seri Indians wade into the water and haul in the plants, hand over hand. The seeds are dried in the sun, then laid on deerskins, cloth or baskets to be threshed with wooden clubs. The grain is tossed into the air to winnow the husks from it. Then it is toasted and pounded to open the tough coats, winnowed again, then ground into flour. The flour was traditionally flavored with sea turtle oil or honey. And the seeds were sometimes eaten with seeds of the *cardon,* a giant cactus.

Modern agronomists tell us that the Green Revolution, which is supposed to feed the world's hungry people in the future, depends on only a few varieties of cereals, carefully bred to produce exactly what the scientist wanted to achieve.

182

As these grains succumb to disease or insect pests, it will be necessary to cross them with older varieties or wilder varieties to renew their vigor. But there are complications.

Charles Heiser in *Seed to Civilization* tells us that there exists a reservoir of potentially valuable genes for use in future breeding programs—the old varieties of plants, the kind which primitive people eat. But new improved, highly-bred varieties are spreading rapidly over the world. And the old varieties are being lost. Seed banks are finally being established to save these older varieties, but much more needs to be done.

Wealthy drug companies are sending specialists to the far corners of the earth searching for exotic plants that may contain substances valuable for the manufacture of drugs. They are aware of the necessity to move fast, for the bulldozers are pushing into remote places at a terrifying speed. Superhighways are being laid down across previously impenetrable jungles.

And not just in jungles. The Pine Barrens Region of Southern New Jersey is the ancestral home of countless plants which are unique to this area. Botanists do not know why they are found only here. As development pushes irrevocably into these pleasant green acres, so close to the mammoth megalopolis of the Northeastern United States, these plants will be lost forever. There is no way to save them once the bulldozers arrive. In every part of the world, as increasing population forces the "development" of more and more land, priceless treasures of undiscovered plant life are disappearing, forever lost to mankind.

We hear a great deal about the many animals which are facing extinction. The same is true of plants. At present it is estimated that some 20,000 plant species will be forever lost if we do not take heroic steps to save them now. As our food situation worsens and hunger stalks more and more millions with every passing year, we cannot afford these losses. In the case of cereals alone, the loss of wild varieties may mean eventual starvation for all of us, for we depend on them for breeding new vigor into our cultivated varieties. It is a situation deserving of a great deal of serious attention from everyone.

Bibliography

√Adams, Ruth and Frank Murray, *The Good Seeds, The Rich Grains, The Hardy Nuts,* Larchmont Books, New York, 1973

Baglin, Douglass, Photography, and Roland Robinson, Text, *The Australian Aboriginal in Colour,* A. H. and A. W. Reed, Sydney, Wellington, Auckland, 1968

Bailey, L. H. *The Standard Cyclopedia of Horticulture,* The Macmillan Company, New York, 1927

Ball, Ian M., *Pitcairn: Children of Mutiny,* Little Brown and Co., Boston, 1973

Balls, Edward K., *Early Uses of California Plants,* University of California Press, Berkeley, Los Angeles, London, 1972

√Banik, Allen E., and Renee Taylor, *Hunza Land,* Whitehorn Publishing Co., Long Beach, California, No date

Bates, Marston, *Where Winter Never Comes,* Charles Scribner's Sons, New York, 1952

Beals, Carleton, *Nomads and Empire Builders,* Chilton Co., Phila. and New York, 1961

Bolton, Ralph, *Aggression and Hypoglycemia Among the Qolla,* "Ethnology," Vol. XII, 1973

Borgstrom, Georg, *Too Many,* The Macmillan Company, New York, 1969

Bray, Warwick, *Everyday Life of the Aztecs,* B. T. Batsford, London; G. P. Putnam's Sons, New York, 1968

Brothwell, Don and Patricia, *Food in Antiquity*, Frederick A. Praeger, New York, Washington, 1969

Buck, Sir Peter Henry, *The Coming of the Maori*, Wellington Maori Purposes Fund Board, distributed by Whitcombe and Tombs, 1952

Cleave, T. L., *Peptic Ulcer*, The Williams & Wilkins Co., Baltimore, Maryland, 1962

Cleave, T. L. and G. D. Campbell, *Diabetes, Coronary Thrombosis and The Saccharine Disease*, John Wright & Sons Ltd., Bristol, England, 1966

Cleland, Herdman Fitzgerald, *Our Prehistoric Ancestors*, Coward McCann, New York, 1928

Coon, Carleton S., *The Hunting Peoples*, Little Brown and Co., Boston, Toronto, 1971

Covarrubias, Miguel, *Island of Bali*, Alfred A. Knopf, New York City, 1937

Drummond, J. C. and Anne Wilbraham, *The Englishman's Food, Five Centuries of English Diet*, Jonathan Cape, London, rev. ed. 1958

Edlin, H. L., *Plants and Man*, Nature and Science Library, The Natural History Press, Garden City, N.Y., 1969

Ehrlich, Paul R., *The Population Bomb*, A Sierra Club-Ballantine Book in paperback, Ballantine Books, New York City, 1968

Everett, T. H., Editor, *New Illustrated Encyclopedia of Gardening*, Greystone Press, New York, MCMLX

Food Composition Table for Use in East Asia, U.S. Department of Health, Education and Welfare, and Food and Agriculture Organization of the United Nations, 1972

Furnas, J. C., *Anatomy of Paradise*, Wm. Sloane Associates, Inc., New York, 1937

Gessler, Clifford, *The Road My Body Goes*, A John Day Book, Reynal and Hitchcock, New York, 1937

Haines, Francis, *The Nez Percé*, University of Oklahoma Press, Norman, 1955

Harrisson, Tom, *Savage Civilization*, Alfred A. Knopf, New York, 1937

Health of the American Indian, U.S. Department of Health, Education and Welfare, DHEW Publication No (HSM) 73–5118, Washington, D.C., 1973

Heiser, Charles B., Jr., *Seed to Civilization, The Story of Man's Food*, W. H. Freeman and Company, San Francisco, 1973

186

Heizer, R. F. and M. A. Whipple, *The California Indians, a Source Book,* University of California Press, Berkeley and Los Angeles, 1960

Hughes, Charles Campbell, *An Eskimo Village in the Modern World,* Cornell University Press, Ithaca, New York, No date

Hunter, Beatrice Trum, *Fermented Foods and Beverages, an Old Tradition,* Keats Publishing, Inc., New Canaan, Conn., 1973

Huxley, Francis, *The Affable Savages,* The Viking Press, New York, 1957

Jekyll, Gertrude and Sydney R. Jones, *Old English Household Life,* Charles Scribners Sons, New York, 1939

Jenness, D., *The Life of the Copper Eskimos,* Johnson Reprint Corporation, New York and London, 1970

Jenness, Diamond, *Indians of Canada,* National Museum of Canada Bulletin 65, Anthropological Series, no. 15

Kahn, E. J., Jr., *The Big Drink, The Story of Coca Cola,* Random House, New York, 1950

Kumlien, Ludwig, *The Natural History of Arctic America, Made in Connection with the Howgate Polar Expedition,* Government Printing Office, Washington, D.C., 1879

Lappé, Frances Moore, *Diet for a Small Planet,* Ballantine Books, New York City, 1971

Latourette, Kenneth Scott, *The Chinese, Their History and Culture,* The Macmillan Co., New York, 4th Printing, 1966

Marshall, Robert, *Arctic Village,* The Literary Guild, New York, 1933

Mowat, Farley, *The Desperate People,* Little Brown and Co., Boston, Toronto, 1959

Murdock, George Peter, *Our Primitive Contemporaries,* Macmillan Co., New York, 1934

Murphy, Margaret A., *The Splendour That Was Egypt,* Philosophical Library, New York, 1951

Oliver, W. H., *The Story of New Zealand,* Roy Publishers, New York City, 1960

Papashvily, Helen and George, *Russian Cooking,* Time-Life Books, New York, 1969

Peterson, Frederick A., *Ancient Mexico,* Capricorn Books, New York, 1962

Prentice, E. Parmalee, *Hunger and History,* Harper and Brothers, New York, 1939

Price, Weston, *Nutrition and Physical Degeneration,* Price-Pottenger Nutrition Foundation, 137 No. Canyon Blvd., Monrovia, California, 1973

Quain, Buell, *Fijian Village,* University of Chicago Press, Chicago, Illinois, 1948

Quennell, Marjorie and C. H. B., *Everyday Life in Prehistoric Times,* G. P. Putnam's Sons, New York, 1959

Radin, Paul, *Indians of South America,* Doubleday Doran and Co., Garden City, N.Y., 1942

Rodale, J. I., *The Healthy Hunzas,* Rodale Press, Emmaus, Pa.

Salzman, L. F., *England in Tudor Times,* B. T. Batsford Ltd., London, 1926

Sameh, Waley-el-dine, *Daily Life in Ancient Egypt,* McGraw Hill Book Co., N.Y., 1964

Simak, Clifford D., *Prehistoric Man, The Story of Man's Rise to Civilization,* St. Martin's Press, N.Y., 1971

Smith, C. Earle, Jr., Editor, *Man and His Foods, Studies in the Ethnobotany of Nutrition—Contemporary, Primitive and Prehistoric Non-European Diets,* The University of Alabama Press, University, Alabama, 1973

Stefansson, Vilhjalmur, *The Friendly Arctic,* The Macmillan Company, New York, 1943

Sweet, Muriel, *Common Edible and Useful Plants of the West,* Naturegraph Company, Healdsburg, California, 1962

Tannahill, Reay, *Food and History,* Stein and Day, New York City, 1973

Tanzer, Helen H., *The Common People of Pompeii, a Study of the Graffiti,* The Johns Hopkins Press, Baltimore, 1939

Taylor, Renee, *Hunza Health Secrets,* Prentice-Hall, Englewood Cliffs, New Jersey, 1964

Thomson, Gladys Scott, *Life in a Noble Household, 1641–1700,* Alfred A. Knopf, New York, 1937

Tobe, John H., *Hunza-Adventures in a Land of Paradise,* Rodale Books, Emmaus, Pa., 1960

Turnbull, Colin M., *The Mountain People,* Simon and Schuster, New York, 1972

Van der Post, Laurens and the Staff and Editors of Time-Life Books, *African Cooking,* Time-Life Books, 1970

Van Valin, William B., *Eskimoland Speaks,* The Caxton Printers,

Caldwell, Idaho, 1941

Verrill, A. Hyatt, in collaboration with Otis W. Barrett, *Foods America Gave the World,* L. C. Page and Co., Boston, 1937

Wallis, Wilson D. and Ruth Sawtell Wallis, *The Micmac Indians of Eastern Canada,* University of Minnesota Press, Minneapolis

Wason, Betty, *Cooks, Gluttons and Gourmets,* Doubleday and Company, Inc., Garden City, N.Y., 1962

Watt, Bernice K. and Annabel L. Merrill, *Composition of Foods, Agriculture Handbook No. 8,* U.S. Department of Agriculture, Washington, D.C., 1963

Weltfish, Gene, *The Lost Universe,* Basic Books, Inc., New York, London, 1965

Weyer, Edward Moffat, Jr., *The Eskimos, Their Environment and Folkways,* Yale University Press, New Haven, 1932

Weyer, Edward Moffat, Jr., *Primitive Peoples Today,* Doubleday and Co., Garden City, No date

Willoughby, Charles C., *Antiquities of the New England Indians,* Harvard University, Cambridge, Mass., 1935

Wolf, Linda, and the Editors of Time-Life Books, *The Cooking of the Caribbean Islands,* Time-Life Books, N.Y., 1970

Yudkin, John, *The Complete Slimmer,* Macgibbon and Kee, London, England, 1964

also in paperback as *Lose Weight, Feel Great,* Larchmont Books, New York City, 1974

Yudkin, John, *Sweet and Dangerous,* Peter H. Wyden Inc. Publishers, New York, 1972

Index